D1461352

16

'1 4 APR

100260828

Work-Related Programs in Occupational Therapy

The *Occupational Therapy in Health Care* series,
Florence S. Cromwell, Editor

Work-Related Programs in Occupational Therapy

Florence S. Cromwell
Editor

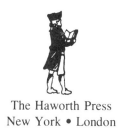

The Haworth Press
New York • London

Work-Related Programs in Occupational Therapy has also been published as *Occupational Therapy in Health Care*, Volume 2, Number 4, Winter 1985/86.

The Haworth Press, Inc., 28 East 22 Street, New York, NY 10010
EUROSPAN/Haworth, 3 Henrietta Street, London WC2E 8LU England

Library of Congress Cataloging-in-Publication Data
Main entry under title:

Work-related programs in occupational therapy.

    "Has also been published as Occupational therapy in health care, volume 2, number 4, winter 1985/1986."
    Bibliography: p.
    1. Occupational therapy—Social aspects. 2. Occupational training. I. Cromwell, Florence S.
RM735.W58   1985   615.8'5152   85-17690
ISBN 0-86656-487-X
ISBN 0-86656-519-1 (pbk.)

Work-Related Programs in Occupational Therapy

Occupational Therapy in Health Care
Volume 2, Number 4

CONTENTS

SOMETHING NEW AND USEFUL . . .

BOOK REVIEWS

DIANE SHAPIRO, MA, OTR, *Director Therapeutic Activities, Department of Psychiatry-Westchester Division, The New York Hospital-Cornell Medical Center, White Plains, NY*

SUSAN L. SMITH, MA, LOTR, FAOTA, *Director, Professional Occupational Therapy Services, Metairie, LA*

LYLA M. SPELBRING, PhD, OTR, FAOTA, *Former Head of Department of Associated Health Professions, Eastern Michigan University, Ypsilanti*

JANET C. STONE, BA, OTR, *Former Department Head, Occupational Therapy, Rancho Los Amigos Hospital, Downey, California, and Initiating Editor, AOTA Bulletin on Practice, Huntington Beach, CA*

CARL SUNDSTROM, MA, OTR, LTC, AMSC, *Occupational Therapy Staff Officer, Health Services Command, Fort Sam Houston, TX*

ELLEN DUNLEAVEY TAIRA, MPH, OTR, *Consultant in Program Development in Long Term Care and Editor,* Physical & Occupational Therapy in Geriatrics, *Kailua, HI*

JENNIFER WAMBOLDT, OTR/L, *Assistant Director, Occupational Therapy, Schwab Rehabilitation Center, Chicago, IL*

MARY GRACE WASHBURN, MHA, OTR, FAOTA, *Marketing Director, Health Care Design Services, Kirkham, Michael and Associates, Architects, Engineers, and Planners, Denver, Colorado*

CARLOTTA WELLES, MA, OTR, FAOTA, *Consultant, Professional Liability, and Former Chairman, Occupational Therapy Department, Los Angeles City College, Los Angeles, CA*

Work-Related Programs in Occupational Therapy

FROM THE EDITOR'S DESK

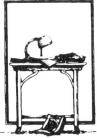

As this issue goes to press, the AOTA Atlanta Conference has just concluded. Given our theme, it was both very exciting to hear there of the burst of interest and development by occupational therapists in work-related programming, and the reinforcement for the potentials for such market and activity which were heard from past-presidents Baum and Hightower-VanDamm. In addition many clinicians on the 'firing line' voiced hope that this arena would offer to them one answer for 'new markets' for occupational therapy services.

As a writer in this issue has said, 'the time is now, the need/demand is out there'. Thus *OTHC* is pleased to present to readers a collection of ideas from writers who know, from the real world, what is happening by and for occupational therapists in the area of work-focused treatment programs.

Unfortunately, one small volume cannot bring the wealth of ideas and interests that occupational therapists are currently demonstrating in this kind of practice, though we do give you live testimony to the vitality and viability of our skills in the changing health care services market. Two issues ago we brought you models of *private practice*[1] which are reiterated here in several papers. However, these work-related treatment activities can be found in *any* of the settings in which occupational therapists find themselves—and can be well integrated into existing 'traditional' programs. Some authors in the current volume feel this kind of programming is better suited

---

[1]*Private Practice in Occupational Therapy,* Vol. 2 #2, Summer 1985. New York: The Haworth Press, Inc.

1

to the community. Whatever the case, the opportunity is now. *AJOT* has recently offered an issue on this same subject;[2] there are also many texts offering now ideas for the uninitiated. We hope you will be inspired and instructed by the material we offer here.

As a tangential, but no less vital arena, the work environment has many dimensions. It was decided to include several papers pertaining to management and leadership concerns in this issue . . . in our *Practice Watch* feature. Significant contributions are offered to persons having or aspiring to those roles of leader and manager. Your attention and comment is invited to this way of augmenting regular thematic content.

In addition, our other feature—*Something New and Useful*—brings information on a work-related assessment now available for use by therapists working with adults with mental retardation. It offers something indeed different from the resources available, typically for working with the young retarded.

Finally, in this issue, we institute a *Book Review* section to offer information on titles related to our theme and content.

Thus ends Volume II of *OTHC*—eight issues and quite a few ideas later from our beginning two years ago. In keeping with our initial goals of offering more *ideas* about practice by more *practitioners,* we have presented 61 papers and features in 4 issues, representing the work of 74 authors, a 20% increase over Volume I in papers, 16% more writers. Who says occupational therapists do not do interesting things *and* share them. Please join us as a contributor. Your ideas are sought and welcome.

Florence S. Cromwell
Editor

---

[2]*American Journal of Occupational Therapy,* Vol. 39, #5 May 1985. Rockville, MD, AOTA.

FROM ANOTHER PERSPECTIVE:
AN OVERVIEW OF THE THEME

Laura Harvey-Krefting, MA, OT(C)

This volume heralds yet another, much needed reawakening of interest in work-related programs. Historically, the theory and philosophy of occupational therapy has strongly supported vocational activity. As Cromwell's review suggests, the potential for occupational therapist has been noted since World War I. In the last decade, numerous writers, myself included, have enthusiastically described work-related therapy as the most promising frontier of practice. And each of the writers in this issue comments on the resurgence of interest in the area. However, in the past this optimism has been followed by a lack of any significant development of work-related therapy. Although much has been written, little action has been taken. Furthermore, this area of practice has stagnated in spite of impetus for growth such as legislation for disabled workers, wars, and technological advances. In order to develop this area of practice we need activities such as; the establishment of a special interest section in the American Occupational Therapy Association (acknowledging the valiant attempts in the past), formulation of models of practice, construction of standardized instruments, and development of a standardized vocabulary.

The writers in this volume revitalize work-related practice. Their

Laura Harvey-Krefting, School of Rehabilitation Medicine, University of British Columbia, and currently in doctoral studies, University of Arizona, Tucson, AZ.

This article appears jointly in *Work-Related Programs in Occupational Therapy* (The Haworth Press, 1985), and in *Occupational Therapy in Health Care,* Volume 2, Number 4 (Winter 1985/1986).

programs are innovative and illustrate viable new roles in health promotion and prevention, private practice, work evaluation, and developmental treatment of adolescents. These therapists go one step further than providing a purely theoretical perspective on the role of occupational therapy in vocational rehabilitation; the "nuts and bolts" descriptions of their programs bring the area to life. However, these papers also illustrate some of the barriers that have prevented work-related occupational therapy from fulfilling its potential.

One of the barriers to the development of work-related occupational therapy is its ambiguous definition both conceptually and in practice. This is clearly illustrated in the variety of terms that are used in this volume to describe the area of practice. Work-related programs, work programming, health care in industry, vocational rehabilitation; each of these labels is descriptive yet the diversity is confusing to patients, referral agents, and to members of the occupational therapy community. This indicates a need for development of and adherence to a common vocabulary to describe the various areas and methods applicable to work-related occupational therapy.

From the theoretical perspective, ambiguity arises with the interchangeable use of the terms vocation and occupation in work-related literature. Occupation is a key construct in our theoretical base yet because of its breadth, it confuses the role of the work-related therapist. For example, do therapists in work-related settings treat homemakers? If one accepts the all-encompassing definition of occupation, and homemaking is the major role of the patient, then, it may be considered work-related treatment. The distinction between these two terms is an important one in overcoming definitional problems. Some agreement on boundaries needs to occur. An example could be defining work-related practice as that which focuses specifically on the employment aspect of productivity, or as Cromwell noted from legislation defining the scope of work-related programs as "return to remunerative employment". The importance of other major life roles, such as the homemaker, student, and hobbyist, need to be acknowledged but considered outside the realm of work-related treatment.

On a more practical level, the diversity of roles and skills that are described in this volume suggest both optimism and confusion. It is difficult to define an area of practice with roles as wide ranging as splint-making for disabled workers, social skills training for special needs adolescents, and leisure counseling for the worker. Moreover, the notion of prevention and promotion in industry adds to the ambiguity of the field. Writers such as Mungai and Bear-Lehman and McCormick describe preventive programs as work-related and therapists are, in fact practicing in the industrial sector. However, many of the activities undertaken in these programs (alcohol and substance abuse counselling, cardiac rehabilitation, and identification of high risk industrial tasks) differ significantly from programs focused on work-related disability. These preventative definitions of work-related practice differ again from that provided by Jacobs et al. in their proactive work therapy for special needs adolescents. Though the variety of opportunity available in work-related settings is encouraging, some accepted definition needs to be applied that will more firmly set the boundaries.

The diversity of potential roles for the occupational therapist can also give a superficial appearance of defining practice by the market place, that is, expanding into areas where health care dollars are available rather than where our expertise is truly applicable. Following the market is useful for development of expertise provided that the new opportunities truly reflect the definition of this area of practice. It is my contention that occupational therapists would benefit from isolating those work-related areas they can best address. Proving ourselves in these areas is critical before diversifying; rapid expansion can dilute the strength of our skills as a profession.

Competition offered by the multitude of other health professionals claiming expertise in the field increases the ambiguity of definition as a barrier to the development of work-related practice. Writers in this volume have identified some of the other professionals as: rehabilitation nurses, counselors, psychologists, engineers, ergonomists, industrial safety managers, work evaluators ad infinitum. It is not surprising that referral agents are perplexed about which professional can best address each work-related problem.

Therapists have long promoted a multi-disciplinary perspective and have been largely successful in working out role boundaries with the other professionals with whom they interact. However, work-related therapy has attracted a vast number of professionals who are competing for the health care dollar devoted to rehabilitation of the worker. Competition in an area that is so ill-defined further increases the risk of losing a place in the work-related arena. Ellexson and Bear-Lehman advocate increased communication between medical centers and industrial settings as a means of working with the disciplines involved in work-related settings. Clearly determining who is best qualified to offer a particular service would foster growth in the area. In addition continued exchange at professional meetings and through journals would help to clarify each profession's boundaries. For work-related practice to succeed we must turn competitive spirit into one of cooperation.

The diversity of roles described in this volume also raises the issue of whether entry level therapists are sufficiently trained to work in this area of practice. Certainly such areas as job analysis, pre-vocational skills, and work simulation are included in the undergraduate curricula but are these sufficient? These writers describe the need for expertise in conducting and interpreting vocational aptitude and interest tests, in work hardening, in job search training, and in ergonomic evaluation. They also refer to the special knowledge needed in dealing with worker's compensation, unions, and the legal profession. But can one more area of knowledge be crammed into the already burgeoning undergraduate curriculum? I think not. What is needed are innovative graduate programs like that proposed by the University of Alberta, in which therapists can build on their basic training and gain confidence in their skills in this very competitive area of practice. In addition, special certification would ensure that those therapists employed in work-related settings, have a similar knowledge base.

These program descriptions do much to advance the image of work-related occupational therapy as an exciting, challenging (and often lucrative) area of practice. Historically, however, it has been somewhat lackluster. Perhaps it has been neglected because of our long allegiance with the medical profession, vocational practice being vaguely related to education of labour, and not really considered "treatment" (certainly not in the same league with the ICU therapist). But in accepting this cloak of respectability and security offered by the medical model, the image of the vocational occupational therapy has suffered. The program descriptions contained in this volume are a first step in improving the image and the visibility of work-related practice. Continued efforts are needed to attract bright and energetic therapists to this field. And there is some urgency in this mission, the longer therapists wait, the tougher the competition we have to face.

This volume presents a challenge for our profession. It lies in maintaining the momentum generated by these papers and ensuring that this multi-faceted, lucrative area of practice develops into a respected specialization in occupational therapy. In discussing what I consider to be the barriers to the development in work-related occupational therapy, I do not intend to paint a dismal future for this area of practice. But it is only in identifying areas critical to the expansion of the field that it will reach its full and rich potential.

Work-Related Programming in Occupational Therapy: Its Roots, Course and Prognosis*

Florence S. Cromwell, MA,OTR, FAOTA

ABSTRACT. This paper presents an examination of the historical evolution of work-related theory in occupational therapy as it paralleled environmental influences (social, political, technical) and how that has affected the thrust and position of the profession today.

Early precursors of occupational therapy as we know it today are found in the history of the care of the mentally ill. As the first humane approaches to treatment emerged in Europe in the late 18th century, they appeared in the form of "work" programs called alternately occupation, activity, industry, ergotherapy. Pinel in France in 1876 first began the use of occupational therapy.

Prescribed physical exercises and manual occupation should be employed in all mental hospitals . . . Rigorously executed manual labor is the best method for securing morale . . . The return of convalescent patients to their previous interests, to the practice of their profession; to industriousness and perseverence have always been for me the best omen of final recovery.[1]

Florence S. Cromwell is Editor of *Occupational Therapy in Health Care.* In addition, she has been long associated with work-focused activity in occupational therapy and has authored several works in this practice area over the years.
*Parts of this article appeared originally in *PIVOT* (Planning and Implementing Vocational Readiness in Occupational Therapy), a curriculum developed by the American Occupational Therapy Association, Rockville, MD, 1985. Edited by Martha Kirkland and Susan C. Robertson.

This article appears jointly in *Work-Related Programs in Occupational Therapy* (The Haworth Press, 1985) and in *Occupational Therapy in Health Care,* Volume 2, Number 4 (Winter 1985/1986).

Our forebears and founders picked up that thread of interest in work in their earliest formulations of the profession's focus and purpose. Adopting "occupation" as the heart of their concerns, they spoke of "work cure" (Hall 1910),[2] "invalid occupations, habit training, handwork occupations including . . . pre-industrial and productive work" (Kidner 1924),[3] by Barton who explained the profession's thrust as "the idea is to give that sort (of activity) which will be preliminary to and dovetailed with the real vocational education which is to begin as soon as the patient is further along" (1919),[4] and by Dunton who felt occupational therapy should "re-establish the patient's capacity for industrial and social usefulness" (1915).[5]

Reviews of both definitions and philosophies and educational strategies in the years since the AOTA was founded continue to reflect the profession's avowed commitment to *work* and work-related activities as distinct parts, if not the core, of occupational therapy. Kielhofner says,

> The concept of work should include all forms of productive activities whether or not they are reimbursed . . . productive activities are those that provide a service or commodity needed by another or that add new abilities, ideas or knowledge, artistic objects or performances to cultural tradition . . . When an activity is considered to be one's work, it is generally organized into a major life role . . . thus activities engaged in to fulfill one's duties as a student, housewife, volunteer, serious hobbyist or amateur (as well as of worker) and that are part of one's identity can be considered work . . . According to this definition work is not limited to adults; it extends to school-age children. Such a broad definition of work is relevant to occupational therapy since many of the field's clients and patients do not have access to marketplace labor.[6]

Thus the door is open for occupational therapists to develop vocational readiness programs. In the context of the Kielhofner definition, there are many possibilities based on the use of occupation in its broadest sense. Occupations can be viewed as the dominant influence on work role success for ill, injured, and disabled people. The actuality of there being such demands in society for this function is, and has consistently been, influenced by many social and political forces.

In order to understand how the concept of vocational readiness programming has evolved through the years, an interlocking review process will be used. This process will (1) explore the relationships and influences of prevailing sociocultural need and action, (including legislative and regulatory mandates), (2) the technological developments in society and health care, and (3) the philosophies and actions of the profession regarding the meaning and use of work-focused activities. Particular points will be made regarding the meeting of needs of handicapped individuals as they were or were not addressed.

SECTION I

Early programs of occupational therapy in the United States were influenced by activities in Europe. Cultural traditions were transplanted from Europe through the colonists. In the early 19th century specific examples related to our theme were recorded.

Moral treatment was widely accepted in the care of the mentally ill in Europe throughout the 1800s. Evidences of occupational therapy-based programs existed in the United States where occupation or work replaced harsh custodial care (Friends Asylum, Philadelphia, 1817; McLean Asylum, Boston, 1818; Bloomingdale Asylum, White Plains, NY, 1821).[7] However, there were not strong moves toward comprehensive or humane care of the ill and disabled in the U.S. until later in the century. The period of 1840 to 1880 marked the highlight of moral treatment and occupational therapy.

The work and writing of Adolph Meyer provided the first philosophy of the incubating profession when he said healthy living involved a "blending of work and pleasure."[8] At about the same time The Industrial School for Crippled and Deformed Children in Boston was established to provide vocational training to disabled children. This was followed by widespread interest in employment opportunities for the handicapped. By 1910 a number of trade schools for "crippled men" and other training workshops for crippled and blind persons had been started.

At this time, the practice of medicine was rudimentary compared with the technology known today. Care of the physically ill was largely palliative involving immobilization and bed rest, and isolation and general removal of patients from all daily roles. Because of such forced idleness, it is not surprising that early occupational therapists became involved in "diversion" activities to create positive mental thoughts and attitudes as well as to break the spells of boredom and inactivity. Vocational readiness programs were rarely seen as pertinent. However, as early as 1913 Herbert Hall, an occupational therapy leader, saw the role of the hospital expanding beyond acute physical care into the realm of vocational training. At his suggestion the Massachusetts General Hospital in Boston started a "workshop" "to fill the dangerous interval . . . immediately after hospital discharge and before regular work can be attempted."[9]

World War I brought more changes. The increased numbers of injured and mentally ill service men and persons injured in industrial accidents required solutions which would get the soldiers back to duty and workers back to their jobs. The Reconstruction Aides (which included occupational and physical therapists), served abroad in France, and in the U.S. provided the first model for occupational therapists as members of a health team.[10] After the war civilian hospitals continued to care for the industrially injured. Probably because of these programs and the significant improvements made in medical care, society began to realize that rehabilitation was a useful concept and should be fostered.

In 1920 the Vocational Rehabilitation Act was passed by the Congress.[11] Through its provisions the foundation for vocational rehabilitation as it is known today was laid. Rehabilitation was defined as "return to remunerative employment" and funds were provided to states on a matching basis for helping disabled persons to that status. The Act allowed solely for "training in existing schools, industry and commercial establishments, or by a tutor." Medical service was covered only "if needed to determine eligibility for help." Carried out by Vocational Education Departments in states, there were many opportunities for occupational therapists in centers such as sheltered and curative workshops to participate in prevocational programming. The extent to which this occurred is not known though some outstanding workshops run by occupational therapists were active in physical and psychological restoration in the period from the 20s and 30s, i.e., the Cleveland Rehabilitation Center, the Milwaukee, Philadelphia, and Delaware Curative Workshops, the St. Louis Workshop, and the Red Cross Institute for the Disabled (later ICD) in New York. By 1938 all 48 states were engaged in rehabilitation programs for the physically disabled.

During this same period, occupational therapists continued to be primary caretakers of the mentally ill. Industrial therapy was an accepted concept in many occupational therapy programs. All patients who were fit were assigned to a job in the operation and maintenance of the facility. The work assignments were based on the belief that "it is possible to teach every patient, aside from senile and paretic cases, some useful occupation which will make them partially or wholly self-supporting and prevent habit deterioration."[12] In many settings occupational therapists were responsible for screening and placing patients as well as for training supervisors and foremen. Activities included every conceivable function, though in general, women were relegated to indoor chores, such as laundry, sewing, kitchen, cleaning, while men worked in maintenance and grounds care as well as in "mechanical" departments.

Concurrently the National Society for the Promotion of Occupational Therapy (later AOTA) moved ahead with professional development based on the agreed focus and definitions of the founding years that "productive occupation as a therapeutic measure" was to "arouse interest, courage and confidence; exercise mind and body in health activities; overcome functional disability and reestablish a capacity for industrial and social usefulness."[13]

In this second statement of the profession's philosophy, return to work roles was again seen as one paramount purpose of occupational therapy. This influence carried to the first educational standards generated in 1923 which included theoretical work designed "to train therapists as teachers of occupations which would help individuals move from acute illness to vocational training."[14] Implicit in this statement is the intent that occupational therapists would be engaged in "work-related" activities if they were to reflect this educational dictum.

The period post-World War I saw the rise of general medicine, and thus the growth of hospitals where occupational therapists were soon caught in the dilemma so often to plague the field in the years ahead, of choosing the "medical" or "vocational" models of care. In the depression years there were still the shared influences and demands on the profession from the two models of care as well as from concern for the disabled. Patients with tuberculosis and chronic disease were widely treated, and persons with cerebral palsy were being recognized as amenable to rehabilitative help. As industry grew, more trauma gave rise to numbers of patients with orthopedic and neurological injuries. Surgery was growing as a medical option.

SECTION II

It was not until the period from 1935-1945 that marked changes occurred in the field. These were brought on by advances in medical care, pharmacology, the wave of social legislation which changed the way Americans would view the aged (Social Security Act, 1935), welfare to the needy, health service agencies, and intensified rehabilitation. PL 113, the Barden LaFollette Act, passed by the Congress in 1943 changed the original provisions of the Vocational Rehabilitation Act of 1920. It did so by providing for medical care to the physically disabled persons seeking vocational assistance and vocational rehabilitation services to the mentally ill as well as to the physical disabled.[15] PL 16 and PL 346 had assured the same coverage for persons with tuberculosis, blindness, industrial injury, and for veterans.[16] A whole wave of rehabilitative activity in health care settings reinforced the concept of returning people to "remunerative employment" as the original definition of rehabilitation decreed.

Industrial therapy continued strongly in psychiatric hospitals, with occupational therapists very active in those programs. No comparable models emerged in institutions caring for persons with other disabilities. Occupational therapists in those settings began to focus on the care of patients with acute illness as well as chronic conditions, largely with "occupation" that was seen as "diversion."

Then came World War II with the enormous increase in demand for rehabilitative services. The military reconditioning programs that resulted were intended to "accelerate return to duty" and incorporated occupational therapy, physical therapy, and speech services. The objective was stated as

> providing for return (of servicemen) to civilian life in the highest possible degree of fitness, well oriented to the responsibilities of citizenship and prepared to adjust successfully to social and vocational pursuits.[17]

Because there were many patients and few occupational therapists, despite war emergency training courses, the focus in military treatment programs was restorative. While some industrial modalities and workshop activities were used as treatment, the essential purpose and focus of programming was on reduction of disability from the acute illness/injury.[18] It was not until the numbers of veterans hospitals rose sharply after the war that more broadly focused programs, including work preparation, appeared. By then, occupational therapists had largely abandoned their interest in work-related programming, deferring to industrial and manual arts "therapists" who were abetted by various counselors. Industrial therapy in all settings was largely eliminated, both by legal decision in response to claims of misuse of patients, and because the emphasis in psychiatric treatment had turned a sharp corner toward psychoanalytic philosophies and techniques.

Occupational therapists in this post World War II decade were engaged in craft activities, which they used interpretively, or as mechanisms for group interaction. This period was the beginning of marked concern for *process* in treatment, more than for content. "Devicing" was the other wave of interest as assistive aids and activities of daily living programs began to dominate treatment concerns. Poliomyelitis, arthritis, burns, hemiplegia, and spinal cord injury presented compelling reasons for attention to immediate self-care needs of patients. Preparation for return to jobs was largely ignored by occupational therapists. At this time, occupational therapy rested within the domain of the medical model. Heightened technology in medicine and the emergence of psychiatric care were major influences in the alliance of occupational therapy with the medical model.

SECTION III

The decade of the 50s provided some startling changes in the care of the severely disabled. These developments stimulated growth in numbers of rehabilitation programs and public interest and support for research concerning the effects of disabling conditions. The August 1954 Amendments to the Vocational Rehabilitation Act, PL 565,(19) was the indication of that public interest.

A specific provision of the 1954 Amendments was the establishment of rehabilitation units in hospitals or rehabilitation facilities to aid in the rehabilitation of disabled persons. Occupational therapists could receive training to provide prevocational evaluation and training. In addition to supplying the funding for research, construction, and scholarships to enhance rehabilitation potentials, the law also drew stronger lines for employment of the handicapped by involving state employment offices. In the same year, there were also changes in Social Security disability provisions which focused public attention on the plight of the disabled worker. The basic and original concept of rehabilitation goals as "return to remunerative employment" continued to prevail, thus sharply limiting the interest in rehabilitation programming (funding) for persons unable or unsuited to such activity. The year 1956 finally saw a change in attitude when "homemaking" was recognized in the regulations as a "vocation" by the U.S. Office of Vocational Rehabilitation.[20] At last broader perspectives so important in considering the needs of the disabled were gaining acceptance.

Schools for handicapped children increased with programs related specifically to the reduction of disability through occupational therapy, physical therapy, and speech services. There is no indication, however, that schools had great concern for the after-graduation lives of the young people. Instead, federal funding led to the expansion of sheltered work opportunities and related prevocational and vocational evaluation services. In these activities occupational therapists were again to assume an important role, and the professional literature in the late 50s and early 60s reflects this activity.[21]

The profession also saw need to "reevaluate" its interest and activity in the area of work-related treatment in the mid-50s. In 1955 a national institute was held to reassess professional education and practice as related to rehabilitation.[21] In 1956 another national institute was convened solely to examine current interest and philosophies related to "prevocational techniques and media." In general the results of the two institutes reflected strong appeal for the potentials for prevocational service in occupational therapy. It was said to be the single most exciting and promising idea facing the profession—a return to engagement in "vocationally related activities in actual treatment and testing situations."[21]

During this same period, occupational therapists in Canada were developing some significant models of vocational readiness programming. This initiative was led by the interests of the Workmen's Compensation Board to hasten return to job of injured workers.[22,23,24,25] Reading of the activities of this period reveals some imaginative approaches used by occupational therapists who gained wide respect for their contributions.

There were other important occurrences during this period that influenced the directions the profession would take over the next 25 years. First, the vocational rehabilitation counseling field was born, with the strong blessing and deliberate support of Mary E. Switzer,

Commissioner of Vocational Rehabilitation.[26] She had spearheaded many legislative activities in the rehabilitation field. Because she saw the need for one specialist to orchestrate the activities required in returning the disabled to productive function, Switzer became a significant leader in the planning and funding of this move. She saw the vocational rehabilitation counselor as the appropriate specialist to carry out the task required. As the field grew, most schools and their students were almost fully subsidized in these early years. Many occupational therapists viewed these specialists as better prepared to evaluate job readiness and to fit persons with disabilities into the right places in employment. Federal funding of rehabilitation programming also supported ever-stronger roles by the vocational rehabilitation counselors. Despite strong encouragement from the federal Office of Vocational Rehabilitation to make occupational therapists more active in prevocational evaluation and training, the profession turned away, because of strong attractions elsewhere.

Most occupational therapists were employed in hospitals where medical technology was expanding rapidly. Polio had been conquered, but there were more patients with severe disabilities, i.e., stroke, arthritis, cerebral palsy, burns, spinal cord injury. Occupational therapists were now drawn to the business of evaluation of function and applying assistive techniques and aids to improve functional daily living skills. The realization that these children and adults needed work role assistance was still not a major concern of occupational therapists, except for preparation of homemakers for their roles. Occupational therapists made significant contributions in the area of functional assessment, and their impact continues to the present day. However, the area of job-readiness became a serious void.

SECTION IV

Through the 60s, the profession appeared to be at a point of indecision and questioning about its future directions. Indecision was evidenced by the self-analysis represented in the Curriculum Study,[27] the Booz, Allen, Hamilton study of association structure and function,[28] and the changing staff patterns in occupational therapy programs resulting from the addition of the assistant level (COTA) to the profession. Some viewed the indecision as a time for a complete change of focus for the profession and its activities. This included more technical and scientific strategies for evaluation and treatment of persons with physical disabilities, a move to community-based psychiatric programming, and a focus on developmental and neurological theory as the fundamental basis for treatment which our founders had espoused. It was also a time when theory development began to be of serious concern to the field.

Rehabilitation as a catch phrase was on the decline. Evidence of occupational therapists' interest and participation in vocational readiness programming was essentially gone. Curative workshops were now comprehensive medical rehabilitation centers. Sheltered workshops were in the hands of business persons who sought contracts, and services were provided by an emerging group of workers called work adjustment or work evaluation specialists who were the product of the federal initiatives which had begun in the mid-50s. The literature of the period records minimal participation by occupational therapists in work programs in the United States.[29] The same was not true in Canada or Europe.

Only one theorist among the leaders of the 60s and early 70s gave any evidence in her research of attention to a global, humanistic approach to care of the disabled as a basis for the profession's activities.[32] There had been no strong iteration of professional philosophy by AOTA since the years of World War II when concern for ''restoration took the lead over return to work'' in occupational therapy programming. A search for an acceptable updated definition of occupational therapy had continued through this decade to no avail. The voices of the field could not find congruence on what was to be the role and image of occupational therapy in the rapidly changing society the United States was experiencing. It was not until 1968 that the annual business meeting finally adopted an official definition of occupational therapy.[30]   In 1979 the Assembly adopted a philosophical base for the profession.[31] In it ''occupation'' was again affirmed as the common core of occupational therapy.

Mary Reilly in 1960[32] published the first of a series of papers in which she introduced her theory of occupational behavior as a compelling basis for education and practice in the profession. In that first paper her now widely quoted injunction, ''Man, through the use of his hands as energized by mind and will, can influence the state of his health,'' became a rallying point for those in the profession who strongly believed productive activity as treatment is the uniqueness and special contribution of occupational therapy. Occupational behavior further asserts that only with balance between work, rest, play, and sleep is healthful living achieved. Work and play lay the basis for the skill acquisition needed through all developmental stages for successful role function. Roles people assume in whatever stage of life, represent their principle activities and arenas for achievement.[33]

Occupational behavior theory offers a return to the concern for occupation, including all forms of productive activity. Thus, the theory speaks to the core of practice as delineated in the 1978 AOTA statement of professional philosophy. Occupational behavior offers a convincing argument for activity or occupation as the major modality of occupational therapy and supports the job of the occupational therapist as actively facilitating all role functions through the use of activity. The therapist using the occupational behavior frame of reference in treatment planning offers a real possibility that the occupational therapist can and will resume a posture in patient care that addresses all work roles with comprehensive use of activities to achieve objectives.

Coincidentally, with AOTA's adoption of the statement of its philosophy for practice, a position paper was prepared on the "Role of the Occupational Therapist in the Vocational Rehabilitation Process" (prepared October 1979, adopted April 1980).[34,35] The paper confirms that practitioners are still actively concerned about work-related treatment. While the paper is a lengthy and detailed exposition of the various functions the occupational therapist offers to persons requiring "vocational rehabilitation services," it does so in a strategy that is oriented to specifically linking the use of occupation as a bridge to work role performance. By inference at least, traditional occupational therapy activities are included in the approaches named. However, the language of this paper is prepared in the mode of vocational rehabilitation and vocational counseling literature and thereby seems to miss the focus of occupation recently reiterated as basic to occupational therapy.

SECTION V

Except for the apparent coalescence of beliefs among practitioners and educators in the philosophical base statement and the updated definition of occupational therapy,[36] the period from 1970 to the present produced little to indicate that work-related treatment by itself is a major focus or concern in the profession. There is now an effort to organize a special interest section in the association to encourage information sharing and program development around work-focused programming.[37] Also there are some significant developments and pockets of interest representing (1) rehabilitation of the injured workman that includes work role evaluation and physical hardening; (2) community based consultative service to industry and insurers regarding placement, training, and/or return of disabled workers to jobs; (3) sheltered or training workshops for the developmentally disabled, learning disabled, and other physically and/or psychologically impaired persons; and (4) career counseling, training, and adjustment programs at community college level for both disabled and language impaired persons. However, no significant percentage of therapists can be said to be involved in these activities. ''Prevocational'' evaluation is still evident in programs in psychiatric settings especially for adolescents. Many of these activities are embraced in living skills programs, which occupational therapists handle ably in both traditional and community based settings.

Accompanying these kinds of activities is a series of significant social legislative acts affecting the disabled and other minority groups. Beginning in 1968 the Architectural Barriers Act[38] led the way to widely felt changes in *access* for disabled people to places and roles that other Americans have enjoyed. The Rehabilitation Act of 1973, followed by amendments, Sections 503 and 504 in 1977,[38] brought many openings for the disabled; the Education for All Handicapped Children Act in 1975 (PL 94-142)[38] made provisions for ''mainstreaming.'' Implementing regulations were not approved until 1977. This concept of servicing for the disabled was met with mixed opinions by educators, parents, and therapists alike. Nonetheless, it is in force, now affecting services to young people to the age of 21. The Educational Amendments of 1976 (Title II—Vocational Amendments),[38] as well as much action directed for services to developmentally handicapped infants, children, and adults, have all had great impact on public attitudes, schooling, and employment potentials and opportunities. Generally more attention is now paid to needs of the disabled overall. Equal opportunity legislation mandated many changes in education and employment access, and in services in general, that affected the disabled along with many others who had been discriminated against. Occupational therapists have been variously involved regionally and locally in the implementation of these laws and regulations, both as service providers and as citizens. The results of these wide-sweeping changes are still evolving. Continuing social change will ultimately spell the results for the disabled as they strive for better and more satisfying role performance.

Nonetheless, the majority of today's practitioners and educators are more active in concerns which directly affect their own function. Educators and practitioners seem almost solely focused on evaluation and treatment strategies for pathology reduction or restoration within the context of medical model rather than the bio-social model that addresses long-range needs of chronically disabled persons in adaptation to role. Those aged, chronically ill, and disabled young individuals currently concentrated in health care facilities will soon be the largest segment of recipients of health care services. The needs of the disabled for independence speak to occupational therapists who can increase their abilities for adapting to role function in work roles . . . the greatest concern and priority of the disabled.

SECTION VI

If occupational therapists accept the challenge and opportunity represented in the needs of the young disabled for better adapted lives despite handicaps, there are critical ways in which occupational therapy personnel should respond. It will require a major shift in thinking about the goals of treatment for handicapped persons as they approach latency and adolescence. The potentials for pathology reduction through treatment strategies now used for handicapped children are minimal except as function is affected by continuing growth and development. More important is a striking change in focus in treatment to attend to the lifelong needs of these chronically disabled people as represented in their work and play roles. During the "student role" years considerable effort should be directed to (1) assisting adaptation to social and occupational roles, (2) building skills and habits for successful living, (3) preparing for the responsibilities of citizenship, and (4) exploring avenues for achievement. Whether these avenues come through hobby, homemaker, volunteer, advocate and/or employee roles, each needs to be addressed with the same care, to lead these young persons through the process of occupational choice[39] by providing the developmental experiences essential to that decision-making step. Here occupation in its fullest context, as described by Kielhofner,[6] is the tool that can bring the greatest potentials for growth and healthy adaptation to work and play roles.

That occupational therapists who now treat people with severe and chronic disability can or will accept such change in emphasis in their treatment planning and implementation depends on the level of commitment the profession demonstrates in the belief that occupation is the uniqueness and power of occupational therapy.

There is a growing number of programs already established and successfully treating people from these perspectives. Therapists in such settings are beginning to speak out and write about their program designs and successes. Disabled adolescents currently in day treatment and residential programs give strong testimony to what can happen with approaches that combine concern for social and cultural influences, lack of skills and abilities for living, as well as inherited or acquired deficit habit structures that seem to defy successful adaptation to life requirements. These are "delinquent," "disturbed," mentally retarded, epileptic adolescents, battered and abused children, or learning disabled youngsters with whom some prior treatment approaches have focused on reduction of their "pathology" rather than on enhancement of their skills. In these occupational behavior oriented settings adapted to normal and usual roles of adolescent and young adult years is the center of interest. Work and play strategies are used to induce change in behavior and in achievement. Healthful patterns of living through learning to balance work, rest, play, and sleep can be taught. Occupation is the catalyst for change.

These kinds of programs and settings offer the greatest potential, and the least chance of perpetuating failure, by addressing the work role potentials of the young disabled in this way.

SUMMARY AND CONCLUSIONS

History of the profession shows us that occupational therapy, its practitioners and its organization through the years, has had a very uneven performance in demonstrating its stated beliefs in "occupation as a matter of prescription"[9] in leading people to happy, productive lives. Further, its participation in programs actually designated as assisting disabled people to "return to remunerative employment," as in the original definition of rehabilitation by the federal Congress,[11] has been spotty.

Both legislative and social forces, including wars, have given impetus to the development of significant examples of programming to assist disabled persons to achieve greater productivity.

The profession through its organization has been consistent in declaring its continuing belief in occupation as central to its function in helping patients achieve healthful living and to "reestablish their capacities for industrial and social usefulness."[5] Only in the past 20 years of the profession's almost 70 years of formalized existence has there seemed to emerge a sound theory that both elucidates and applies the beliefs of the founders, in the context of today's demands. Further, this theory lends promise that the field might embrace its tenets and begin to develop programs around the humanistic goals originally verbalized by founders under the rubric of occupational behavior.

Fundamental in any case is the concern that occupational therapy programming to assist young disabled people to acquire the skills and habits they will need for successful adaptation in a highly technical society must begin. A change in focus from pathology reduction to facilitating the acquisition of work and play skills is a good beginning. These skills can lead to achievement and role success so essential to the adjustment and productivity of any human, disabled or not.

REFERENCES

Introduction Section

1. Pinel P: medical philosophical treatise on mental aberration, in Licht, S: *The Occupational Therapy Source Book.* Baltimore: Williams and Wilkins Co, 1948, chap 7

2. Hall H J: Work cure, a report of five years experience at an institution devoted to the therapeutic application of manual work. J A M A 1910:54:12

3. Kidner T B: Reconstruction schemes in hospitals for mental and nervous diseases. *Arch Occup Ther* 1924:3(2):117-120

4. Barton G: *Teaching the Sick: A Manual of Occupational Therapy Re-Education.* Philadelphia: W B Saunders Co, 1919

5. Dunton W: *Occupational Therapy: A Manual for Nurses.* Philadelphia: W B Saunders Co, 1915

6. Kielhofner G: Occupation, in Hopkins H L and Smith H D: *Occupational Therapy* ed 6. Philadelphia: J B Lippincott Co, 1983, chap 3

Section I

7. Licht S: *The Occupational Therapy Source Book.* Baltimore: Williams and Wilkins Co, 1948

8. Meyer A: As quoted in Hopkins H L and Smith H D: *Occupational Therapy,* ed 6. J B Lippincott Co, 1983

9. Hall H J: *A New Profession.* Concord, Mass: Rumford Press, 1923

10. Reed K and Sanderson, S: *Concepts of Occupational Therapy.* ed 2. Baltimore: Williams and Wilkins Co, 1983, p 213-215

11. Rubin S E and Roessler, R T: Foundations of the Vocational Rehabilitation Process, ed 2. Baltimore: University Park Press, 1983

12. Reid E C: Ergotherapy in the treatment of mental disorders. *Bos Med Surg J* 1914: 121(8): 301

13. Dunton W R: Occupational Therapy in *Barr's Modern Medical Therapy in General Practice,* Vol 1. Baltimore: Williams and Wilkins Co, 1940

14. Hopkins H L and Smith H D: *Occupational Therapy,* ed 6. Philadelphia: J B Lippincott Co, 1983

Section II

15. Rubin S E and Roessler R T: *Foundations of the Vocational Rehabilitation Process.* Baltimore: University Park Press, 1983

16. Willard H S and Spackman C S: *Principles of Occupational Therapy,* ed 2. Philadelphia: J B Lippincott Co, chap 6

17. U.S. Government Printing Office, *Occupational Therapy,* War Department Training Manual. Washington, DC 1944

18. West W L: Professional Services of Occupational Therapists, World War II, chap 9. *Army Medical Specialists Corps,* Editors: Lee H S and McDaniel, M L. Washington, DC: Office of the Surgeon General, Department of the Army, 1968

Section III

19. Rubin, #15, op cit

20. Zimmerman, M E: *Occupational Therapy in the ADL Program.* Willard and Spackman, ed 3

21. West W L: role of Occupational Therapy in work Adjustment, in *Work Adjustment as a Function of Occupational Therapy.* Dubuque, IA: Wm C Brown Co, 1963

22. Hood M: Occupational therapy—work tests and assessment. *Can J Occ Ther* 1956, 23 (2)

23. LeVesconte H P: Some aspects of rehabilitation in Canada. *Can J Occ Ther* 1955, 22 (2)

24. Smith H V: Workmen's compensation board, occupational therapy workshop. *Can J Occ Ther,* 1940, 7 (1)

25. Storms, H D: Occupational therapy in the treatment of industrial casualties. *Can J Occ Ther,* 1943, 10 (2)

26. Sussman M B: *Sociology and Rehabilitation.* New York: American Sociological Association, 1966

Section IV

27. *The Curriculum Study.* New York: American Occupational therapy Association, 1963

28. *Study of the American Occupational Therapy Association.* Report to the Executive Board, Booz, Allen and Hamilton Co, 1963

29. Fry R R(ed): *Work Evaluation and Adjustment: An Annotated Bibliography, 1947-77.* Menomonie, Wisc, Stout State Rehabilitation Institute, University of Wisconsin-Stout, 1978

30. Minutes of the Annual Meeting. *Am J Occ Ther,* 1969: 23:185

31. Representative Assembly minutes. *Am J Occ Ther,* 1979: 33:781

32. Reilly M: Occupational therapy can be one of the great ideas of 20th century medicine. *Am J Occ ther* 1962: 16:29

33. Matsutsuyu J: Occupational behavior approach, in Hopkins H L and Smith H D: *Occupational Therapy,* ed 6. Philadelphia: J B Lippincott Co, 1983 chap 8

34. *The Role of the Occupational Therapist in the Vocational Rehabilitation Process.* A Position Paper, American Occupational Therapy Association, April 1980

35. *Reference Manual of the Official Documents of the American Occupational Therapy Association,* 1983

Section V

36. Representative Assembly minutes. *Am J Occ Ther,* 35, 798

37. Jacobs K, Chr and Ed, *Prevocational Group Newsletter.* Andover, MA, 1983

38. Cromwell F S: Know and use current federal legislation. Nationally Speaking Column, *Am J Occ Ther,* 33 (2)

39. Ginzberg E et al.: *Occupational Choice: An Approach to a General Theory.* New York: Columbia University Press, 1961

Vocational Evaluation in the Private Sector: An Occupational Therapy Approach

Patricia C. Smith, MS, OTR
Julie S. Bohmfalk, MS, OTR

ABSTRACT. There is a resurgence of interest in vocational rehabilitation among occupational therapists as evidenced by the number of vocational evaluation programs which have been established in recent years using various models of practice.

This paper will describe the process for practice in a private, freestanding facility in which occupational therapists provide a variety of work related services.

The focus will be on evaluation which is the primary service and usually serves as the keystone to subsequent courses of action.

Occupational therapy has traditionally always been concerned with worker role acquisition and function. A brief search of the health care or vocational rehabilitation literature reveals a long history of occupational therapy in work-focused treatment.[1] The domain of vocational rehabilitation is now enjoying a resurgence of interest among occupational therapists. Whether this comes in response to threatened reimbursement in traditional settings or growing interest in entrepreneurial activities, many vocational evaluation programs have been established by occupational therapists in recent years.

There is a wide assortment of approaches and models by which occupational therapy services are being offered now in this growing specialty area. One will be the focus of the paper to follow. It is *Oc-*

Patricia C. Smith is Director and a Certified Vocational Evaluator (CVE), and Julie S. Bohmfalk is Senior Associate, Occupational Assessment & Modification, 10601 S. DeAnza Blvd. Suite 103, Cupertino, California 95014.

This article appears jointly in *Work-Related Programs in Occupational Therapy* (The Haworth Press, 1985) and *Occupational Therapy in Health Care,* Volume 2, Number 4 (Winter 1985/1986).

cupational Assessment and Modification (OAM), a private-practice facility in northern California. The goal of OAM is to combine the best of comprehensive vocational evaluation and training services along with applications of traditional occupational therapy approaches and expertise in providing environment or equipment modifications, work-related orthotics, adaptive/compensatory techniques and more.

THE SETTING

Occupational Assessment and Modification is a private practice, free standing facility established to assist people who because of injury or disability need help in assuming or resuming worker roles. Situated in an urbanized area of northern California where high technology development and manufacturing is widespread, the facility draws clients from that sector and from the usual mix of urban service businesses and adjacent agricultural and heavy manufacturing industries.

The clients served represent a diverse population of workers of all ages and educational levels including many highly skilled professional/technical workers. Referrals come primarily from private industrial insurance through their qualified rehabilitation representatives—a role which might, for example, be filled by a vocational rehabilitation counselor. The majority of referrals are for vocational evaluation, but also include referrals for doing job analyses, determining needs for adaptive aids for job function, home or job-site modifications to improve or make possible specific tasks, dominance retraining and work hardening programs before return to regular job demands.

The facility and its staff interface regularly with a number of other disciplines, from insurance, law, medicine, special education, vocational counseling, business and industry. These other service disciplines span all phases of a client's needs from new injury to termination of rehabilitation services. The variety of services clients receive demands that OAM staff be familiar with and responsive to the many needs and constraints (economic, legal, informational) that such a service complex presents. At the same time this facility must provide comprehensive, yet cost and time effective services which capitalize on the strengths of the staff, occupational therapists with graduate degrees and further training and experience in vocational programming and testing. Consultants on the staff include psychologists and a rehabilitation engineer. These consultants provide additional client services as needed.

BASIS FOR SERVICES OFFERED

As the mission statements for the facility were being developed, at the time of organization, it became apparent that a specific practice process, based on a definite theoretical framework, was needed. The theoretical base chosen of OAM originated in the dominant approaches of occupational therapy theory[2,3,4,5] but is augmented from the fields of career education, special education and psychology. Ideas of theorists of such as Super, who described the human development continuum in terms of vocational development,[6] and Brolin and Carver, who have described a model of lifelong career development for handicapped adults[7] have been integrated. The model of human occupation now used at OAM incorporates relevant theories from other disciplines regarding vocational development with occupational therapy theory into a comprehensive model of practice. It has served well as a basis for developing services; it acknowledges the needs of the marketplace, provides accountability in a human service area fraught with litigation and changing regulatory requirements, serves best interests of the disabled client, and helps to advance the competitive position of occupational therapists in this growing area by evincing their unique suitability to provide such services.

THE PROCESS

When a client is referred he is scheduled initially for an intake interview. That interview, lasting approximately one hour, routinely includes not only an orientation to the evaluation process in general, but also a medical 'self-report' and a review of perceived physical abilities and limitations. Also undertaken at this time is both a vocational and avocational history with emphasis on identifying skills which might be transferable, a review of relevant social, family and economic circumstances bearing on present client needs, and an exploration of the client's perceived stressors as well as his vocational goals. Finally, from the start in this initial interview, the client is encouraged to become an active participant in the evaluation process and in whatever other services are to follow.

Individual Evaluation Plan

Immediately following the intake interview, staff develop an Individual Evaluation Plan (IEP) for the client. Contributing to it are reviews of relevant medical reports, requests in the referral, information gained in the intake interview, and vocational reports, if available. These collected data provide the basis for developing objectives for further evaluation and for the methods by which those objectives will be met. A formal IEP is required by many regulatory and certifying bodies, and is designed to assure that quality services are rendered. It also facilitates the necessary coordination of effort when more than one evaluator is to be involved with the client, brings focus to the evaluation procedure, and ensures that sufficient pertinent data are collected to respond, within the time allotted for the client, to the specific requests in the referral. The plan provides the basis for delivery of all subsequent services.

FURTHER ASSESSMENT

Physical Tolerances

Concerns for physical abilities and limitations are a frequent basis for referral. Therefore, assessment of such physical attributes begins during the initial interview through observation of movement behaviors such as those in walking, sitting and in use of hands. During that initial interview the client is asked to talk about his abilities and limitations as he perceives them. Assessment of those abilities continues throughout the evaluation period, directly, as the client is involved with tasks in situational and work sample testing designed for the purpose, and indirectly, during psychometric testing and in other encounters with staff.

Most of the physical traits specified for given jobs by the U.S. Department of Labor in the *Dictionary of Occupational Titles*[8] are objectively assessed using standardized testing equipment and other clinical tools. Physical capacities that are specifically affected by given disabling conditions are the main focus of continuing evaluation as the client functions in carefully designed job tasks. Information concerning physical capacities alone, however, is of little benefit to the referral source, or may even be misleading, if other factors affecting performance and employment are not also assessed and reported.

Work-Related Behaviors

Fundamental to a comprehensive evaluation of the injured worker is a careful assessment of work-related behaviors. Basic education and training of occupational therapists qualifies them to use interviews and standardized tests, as well as observation, to gather and report subjective and objective data on patient performance, including that which pertains to worker behaviors. Nonetheless, occupational therapists are frequently limited in knowledge or use of tests of achievement and of vocational interests and aptitudes. Most occupational therapists, therefore, must add to their basic assessment foundation further knowledge of vocational tests, their selection, administration and interpretation, in order to be well prepared to evaluate and report performance in the areas critical to worker performance.

Frequently, there are purchase and use requirements for many of the tests which are most suitable to vocational assessment. Requirements often include demonstrating completion of advanced level course work in testing (or equivalent training) if one is to administer tests without supervision of other 'qualified' personnel. This can present a serious roadblock to occupational therapy vocational programming.

At OAM, assessment of worker behaviors is a fundamental part of a total evaluation. Most psychometric instruments are administered and interpreted by the occupational therapists/evaluators. Those requiring administration and interpretation by a licensed psychologist are done by consulting staff.

Traditional Occupational Therapy Services in Worker Evaluation

The occupational therapy process used at OAM offers through its broad scope the flexibility for staff to incorporate a wide array of work-related services usual to occupational therapy. These include such things as adapting tools, giving specific training in body mechanics for certain jobs or tasks, offering dominance retraining for the worker with an injured dominant hand, and training workers in techniques which help them to compensate for performance losses. All these are integral parts of worker rehabilitation. Vocational evaluation in an occupational therapy facility is not a 'medical' treatment performed in a 'medical' setting. Traditional occupational therapy services, however, in this context, may consist of 'treatment' techniques appropriate and necessary to prepare an individual for job performance. The referral sources are made aware of such services, their costs and time requirements through public relations and marketing efforts. Goals for *all* services are always vocationally related.

The following are some examples of worker related services which OAM provides on request, either as part of the evaluation or in subsequent services. Job analyses may be performed on-site to identify job hazards or overcomplex methods, and modifications may be recommended for changing how a job is done, the work site itself or tools and equipment the worker uses. Coordination by the occupational therapist in such efforts with employers/supervisors, corporate officers, payment sources, rehabilitation engineers (if needed) or other interested parties is essential to make certain that recommendations are understood and accepted.

Assistive devices and other orthotics may be designed and fabricated or procured by the occupational therapist, and use training provided to assure the worker's ability to perform on the job successfully. Many of these kinds of services are implemented under the direction of the evaluating occupational therapist. Others must be ordered with physician approval, and require that related documentation be secured and completed by the therapist.

Work hardening, a service which is designed to increase physical ability to handle the demands of work and to promote appropriate worker behaviors, is also offered and may be recommended.

PRESENTING THE RESULTS

The evaluation procedure concludes with an exit interview attended by the injured worker, the person who referred the worker, and the evaluator in which results of the evaluation and their implications for future employment are discussed. The person who referred the worker also receives a report which is a narrative description and analysis of findings written in language free of jargon. It includes the evaluator's recommendations to assist in successful return to employment.

CONCLUSION

In today's climate of worker rehabilitation the evaluator's role is pivotal in making determinations on issues vital to both the client and his referral source. These include feasibility for employment or re-employment, practicality for training or re-training, choices of workable vocational goals, and identification of and arrangement for appropriate training and work environments. In the intense and relatively lengthy association between therapist and client in evaluation, a client reveals much about his behavior, abilities, deficits, motivations and self-image as well as his physical and mental capacities. A large and rich amount of information critical to work success is made available to the alert and sensitive evaluator. Analyzed and translated into vocationally relevant conclusions and recommendations, and presented in a clear and concise way,[9] the efforts of the occupational therapist/vocational evaluator can lay the groundwork for sound and productive worker rehabilitation.

SUMMARY

A free-standing private practice devoted to vocational evaluation and training has been described. Using a strong theoretical base for selecting and implementing services, the practice process at OAM responds to contemporary demands in human services and provides a broad-based, comprehensive service to injured workers. The steps in the process used have been discussed. It is hoped that such a model of service as this may prove useful to other occupational therapists who are or wish to function in work-related programming.

REFERENCES

1. Smith PC, McFarlane B: A work hardening model for the 80's. *Proceedings of the National Forum on Issues in Vocational Assessment,* Menomonie, Wisconsin: Material Development Center, 1984

2. Kielhofner G, Burke JP: A model of human occupation, part 1. Conceptual framework and content. *Am J Occup Ther* 34: 572-581, 1980

3. Kielhofner G: A model of human occupation, part 2. Ontogenesis from the perspective of temporal adaptation. *Am J Occup Ther* 34: 657-663, 1980

4. Kielhofner G: A model of human occupation, part 3. Benign and vicious cycles. *Am J Occup Ther* 34: 731-737, 1980

5. Kielhofner G, Burke JP, Igi CH: A model of human occupation, part 4. Assessment and intervention. *Am J Occup Ther* 34: 777-788, 1980

6. Zaccaria: *Theories of Occupational Choice and Vocational Development,* Boston: Houghton Mifflin, 1970

7. Brolin DE, Carver JT: Lifelong career development for adults with handicaps: a new model. *J Career Education* June, 1982

8. U.S. Department of Labor: *Dictionary of Occupational Titles,* Washington, D.C.: U.S. Government Printing Office, 1977

9. Smith P, Bohmfalk JB: How to improve professional reporting of work evaluations. *Occup Ther in Health Care* 1: 109-114, 1984

The Unique Role
of Occupational Therapy
in Industry

Melanie T. Ellexson, OTR

ABSTRACT. Experienced occupational therapists have five particular characteristics gained from their education and clinical experience which make them uniquely suited for a major role in rehabilitation of persons with industrial injuries. These are: (1) knowledge of injury and illness, (2) understanding of psycho-social aspects of disability, (3) knowledge of the rehabilitation system, (4) ability to analyze tasks and (5) ability to creatively adapt the physical environment. Skills in administration, teaching and the ability to deal with a variety of people from different backgrounds: educational, socioeconomic and work ethic are also vitally important for effective functioning in and with industry.

For the aspirant, the beginning steps are to become familiar with the tasks workers perform, to sell management personnel on a rehabilitation philosophy by showing them how return on investment can be realized, and to inform supervisors, union officials and employees of the goals of such ideas and how they will work in their company.

This paper will describe how one occupational therapist has developed a program and functioned successfully in and with the railroad industry. Analysis of statistics and a case study will show cost savings and return on energy and on initial investment.

The historical link between occupational therapy and industry gives credence to the unique contribution of occupational therapy and establishes the need for more occupational therapists in industry.

Melanie T. Ellexson is a graduate of the University of Illinois Curriculum in Occupational Therapy, has done graduate work in Health Services Administration at Governors State University, University Park, IL, currently lives in Glenwood IL. She is a member of AOTA, IOTA, and American Women in Transportation.

Acknowledgement is made to Lillian Hoyle Parent, MA, OTR, FAOTA for her support, encouragement, and sharing of information, time, and resources.

This article appears jointly in *Work-Related Programs in Occupational Therapy* (The Haworth Press, 1985) and *Occupational Therapy in Health Care,* Volume 2, Number 4 (Winter 1985/1986).

35

In 1922 Adolph Meyer proposed the work-play-rest-sleep continuum emphasizing that the balance between each of these activities was a legitimate concern of occupational therapy.[1] Clare Spackman has stated that "the unique contribution of occupational therapy is that it uses a program of normal activity to aid in the psychological adjustment of the patient, as specific treatment or as a simulated work situation. Thus, it relates to the patient's everyday life and provides the link between hospitalization and return to the community."[2]

It is this link between disability and ability that Florence Cromwell was talking about when she said, " . . . most persons interested in helping the disabled will agree that the beginning of the process, physical and/or mental restoration . . . and the final step, placement in a productive situation . . . are clear cut. The middle step is the difficult one to delineate."[3]

Leaders in occupational therapy have identified this link, this middle step, as being partly the domain of the occupational therapist. This author feels that the occupational therapist can provide valuable aid especially in the rehabilitation of persons with industrial injuries.

The experienced occupational therapist gains five basic qualifications in her education, training and clinical experience which makes her uniquely suited for a major role in industrial rehabilitation. These are:

1. knowledge of injury and illness
2. understanding of the psycho-social aspects of disability
3. knowledge of the rehabilitation system
4. ability to analyze tasks
5. ability to creatively adapt the physical environment

The need for one to have additional skills in administration, instruction/teaching and in dealing with a wide range of people from different educational, socio-economic and work ethic backgrounds will become apparent as the occupational therapists develops her role in this environment.

This paper will describe the role an occupational therapist has developed within the railroad industry, delineating the essential background one must have and the kinds of programs in which one may be involved. A case study will illustrate typical function.

BACKGROUND

In many industrial roles the individual worker is expected by supervisors to be able to do 100 percent of his job. Industry's number one concern is production. Get the job done as quickly as possible using as few individual workers as possible. This is how profit is made. Therefore, it is financially important to bring injured employees back to work as quickly as possible. This stabilizes production, saves costs of training new workers and reduces the company's liability or claim payout. To be effective in planning a rehabilitation program in such settings the occupational therapist must be thoroughly familiar with the potential treatment outcomes and expected physical restrictions at all stages in the recovery from typical injuries found in the setting.

As an example, it would be important to know that a collateral ligament knee injury generally results in some knee instability. In many industries this may mean a major job change because the individual can no longer safely climb, walk on uneven surfaces, get on or off moving equipment or stand for long periods of time. Conversely, a meniscus knee injury does not usually result in instability and the person could probably return to full duties.

Based on such understandings and knowledge of the industry involved, the occupational therapist must begin planning a program by teaching management personnel how and why it is to their advantage to allow temporarily or permanently restricted employees to return to work even if some job modification is necessary. In addition, the employee will have to be convinced of the advantages of early return to his job. There are many secondary gains which discourage injured employees from wanting to return to work. They are afraid of re-injury, afraid of their co-workers' reactions and afraid of disciplinary action which frequently follows return from an industrial injury. Since the injured employee is paid for his time off through Workers Compensation or disability insurance, he can also look forward to an additional cash award for his 'pain and suffering'.

Those in the medical community frequently encourage patients in their disability. Let's look at a typical pattern. An injured worker sees an acute care physician who typically orders 'rest', medication and therapy. The 'rest' serves to further the disability by allowing general weakness to develop and by encouraging an invalid role. Medications frequently cause drowsiness, lethargy and may have unpleasant side effects such as nausea. Therapy, of whatever kind, although of some help, draws attention to the injury and contributes to the dependent role. In addition, the injured person may get more attention and special consideration from family members during this time.

Such a pattern is usually perpetuated until one of three things happens:

1. the employee gets better and returns to work despite the prior deterrents to wellness
2. he requires surgery and further dependency
3. the employee becomes chronically disabled.

For the employee who gets better and returns to work it often means that the month or two of sitting around and being dependent and cared for makes his successful return to work difficult as he is now expected to be totally independent and to return immediately to heavy work loads. It is obvious that under such conditions re-injury can occur.

BEGINNING STEPS

The occupational therapist must work with first line supervisors to help them understand these problems and the need to establish realistic work tasks for the gradual re-entry of the individual into the work force. The occupational therapist must also have developed a relationship with the employee to provide an on-going support system for him during this transition. Bringing the employee into the decision-making as to what tasks he will or will not be required to perform, and setting up time frames for different levels of function until return to full duty with the supervisor and the physician is most advantageous. Such structured plans set limits on what the employee can do and give the supervisor realistic expectations of what work can be accomplished. It also indicates to the physician that attention is being given to the continued recovery of his patient. In a case such as this, the occupational therapist has been required to use knowledge of injury and illness, of psycho-social aspects of disability, of task analysis and possibly of environmental (worksite) adaptation, along with instructional, administrative and communication skills to bring about a successful return to work.

THE WORKER NEEDING FURTHER TREATMENT

An individual who does not return to work after a relatively short period of time may proceed either to specialized care in which surgery is frequently indicated, or he may remain in the 'rest, medication and therapy' pattern without significant improvement until he becomes chronically disabled or is labeled as a chronic pain sufferer. This kind of outcome is often the case with patients having the 'number one' industrial injury, low back strain. In these circumstances the occupational therapists' knowledge of the rehabilitation system can be of vital importance because of the complexity of needs of such patients.

In planning for patients with low back conditions it may be necessary for the occupational therapist to encourage the physician to break the pattern of pain and limitation by one of several plans: returning the person early to a restricted job situation, encouraging his transfer to an active daily rehabilitation program at a rehabilitation facility, or seeking referral for the patient to a center offering treatment for chronic pain. In the last two of these situations, the occupational therapist's knowledge of what happens and what can be accomplished in a rehabilitation center or chronic pain facility can be used to encourage the patient and his family to participate. As a representative of both the medical community and industry, it is important for the occupational therapist working in industry to develop good working and active participant roles with all facilities utilized for rehabilitation services. It may also be necessary to assist them in developing programs which are specific to the needs of injured employees.

More and more programs are being developed in major institutions offering rehabilitation services for injured employees unable to return even to restricted jobs. Programs are designed to provide structured daily activity. The individual may receive occupational therapy, physical therapy, psychological and vocational counseling, as well as work adjustment training and safety instruction. Such programs are designed not only to help alleviate a person's physical problems, but also to encourage activity and build endurance. Activity and daily routine can be most critical in preventing chronic disability which tends to develop quickly for persons in inactive programs typical of accepted treatment.

Even if a patient has been through an active rehabilitation or chronic pain program as described previously, the occupational therapist starting a rehabilitation program within a company must go through the same steps developing structured return-to-work routines. For some workers with more serious injury resulting in permanent disability it may be necessary to identify and develop permanent job/task adaptations (accommodations) or a total job change either within or outside of the former company/industry. In making such changes a vocational counselor or a work evaluator can work with the occupational therapist in directing in-house job change or adaptation or in helping the worker to find successful return to work in jobs elsewhere.

DEVELOPING A REHABILITATION PROGRAM IN THE RAILROAD INDUSTRY

"Occupational therapy is based upon the fundamental belief that engagement in purposeful activity (occupation), including both its interpersonal and environmental dimensions, can prevent or remediate dysfunction and elicit maximum performance in work role 'adaptation'."[4] With this in mind, the author developed the first rehabilitation program at a major midwestern railroad company in the fall of 1979. Top management personnel had recognized that recent laws governing the employment of the handicapped, along with soaring medical, legal and claim costs presented problems that had to be addressed and controlled. The first program was started in the Milwaukee area in a locomotive and freight car shop where approximately 1,000 men were employed. Injuries in that shop were about 450 per year, with an average of 2,000 lost work days per year. These figures included only injury and lost time due to on-duty accidents.

After seeking support and cooperation from top management personnel in the company, management people in the repair shops were contacted to explain that with help from an occupational therapist, a program was to be started in which injured employees would be allowed to return to work with restrictions on their job functions. The reception to such an announcement was less than cordial. 'Work at full capacity or don't work at all' had been the rule and change was not a popular idea. There were immediate concerns about production losses, possible increased liability and the lowering of morale generally. Fortunately, with top management support, the program did proceed.

The first change effected was to alter the term 'light duty' to 're-stricted duty'. Light duty cannot be defined; however, work with specific restrictions is a tangible concept. Next, supervisors were asked to aid in the development of a 'health status' form which could easily be completed by physicians and easily understood by first line supervisors. See Figure A. This set forth the restrictions applicable to work assignments.

The next step was to set up a series of meetings with local union chairmen to explain the program and point out the financial benefit to both injured employees and the company. The officials were skeptical and reiterated the position of Labor generally that an em-ployee is the best judge of how he feels and when he can work; therefore, no one should work unless he is 100 percent. It was ex-plained that government regulations would eventually mandate these types of programs. Further, it was stated that steps to reduce lost time and money were crucial to the survival of the company. Local officials were given material outlining details of the program as it benefitted employees and did receive encouragement to cooperate from the general chairmen of their organizations.

Personnel in the medical facilities used by the company were pro-vided with the forms along with a thorough explanation of the pro-gram and its goals. Physicians were assured that all restricted em-ployees would be closely monitored to protect their recovery and to prevent re-injury. Next, the first line foremen were given classroom instruction on the program in which the disability of pain and the psychology of injury were stressed, along with their roles in the pro-gram's success. The emphasis was on primary prevention as well as on the supervision of injured workers. Five categories of workers who have potential for work/job injuries were discussed:[5]

1. The older worker who can no longer sustain a fast pace, who may be counting the days to retirement and who may not have his attention fully focused on his job,
2. The new employee who does not really like or understand what he is doing,
3. The employee who has had his assignment or job changed and is unhappy or unfamiliar with the new tasks,
4. The employee who has gone through or is going through a di-vorce, loss of a parent, child or spouse, or who is living through some other major stress producing incident in his life,
5. The 'hop-scotch worker' who is defined as 'the accident look-

Figure A.

HEALTH STATUS REPORT

		TIME IN_____ AM/PM
TREATMENT AUTHORIZATION: _____		TIME OUT_____ AM/PM
	(Supervisor's Signature)	
Date:_____	Location:_____	

Employee: _____ SSA No. _____ Date:_____

Address: _____ City: _____ Zip: _____ Phone: _____

DIAGNOSIS: _____

PATIENT'S STATEMENT OF WHAT OCCURRED: _____

DATE OF INJURY: _____ DATE OF FIRST TREATMENT: _____

TREATMENT: _____

MEDICATIONS: (Names, Dosages, Contra-Indications) _____

MAY RETURN TO WORK: Full Duty ☐   Restricted Duty ☐   No Work ☐   Estimated time off:_____

RESTRICTIONS:

LIFTING/CARRYING:	Light (10 - 25 lbs.)	☐	NO WORK INVOLVING:	Hand:	R	L
	Moderate (25 - 50 lbs.)	☐		Arm:	R	L
	Heavy (50 + lbs.)	☐		Leg:	R	L
BENDING/STOOPING:	Light (0 - 6 times/hr.)	☐				
	Moderate (6 - 10 times/hr.)	☐	WEAR SPLINT: ☐			
	Heavy (10 + times/hr.)	☐				
PUSHING/PULLING:	Light (10 - 25 lbs.)	☐	SITTING JOB ONLY: ☐			
	Moderate (25 - 50 lbs.)	☐	NO OVERHEAD WORK: ☐			
	Heavy (50 + lbs.)	☐	NOT TO OPERATE MOVING MACHINERY: ☐			
CLIMBING:	No Vertical Ladders	☐	NOT TO GET ON/OFF MOVING TRAINS: ☐			
	No Stairs	☐				
	No Ramps	☐				

REMARKS: _____

DURATION OF RESTRICTIONS: _____

NEXT APPOINTMENT: Date:_____ Time:_____

THERAPY APPOINTMENT(S): Date(s)_____ Time:_____

DATE OF DISCHARGE FROM CARE: _____

_____ MD   Address:_____ Phone:_____
(Signature)   City:_____ Zip:_____

I hereby authorize the above facility to release any and all Medical Information pertaining to the injury described above:

Employee's Signature:_____ Date:_____

Address:_____

City:_____ State:_____ Zip:_____ Phone:_____

PDM 605 REV. 2/83

MEDICAL SERVICES

ing for a place to happen'. This employee is always in the wrong place at the wrong time and continually fails to follow instructions. He has an excuse for everything and is never at fault.

Steps for assisting successful return to work after injury were stressed with supervisors:[5]

1. Early and frequent contact between the first line supervisor and the injured employee should be maintained.
2. Recognize that the person who has been inactive, even for short periods of time, cannot be expected to perform 100 percent of potential immediately.
3. Set limits on activity while adhering to specific allowances and restrictions. Be firm but understanding in instructing workers in what they can do.
4. Avoid harassment of workers who may be uneasy and 'testy'. Keep cool. Testing of authority may occur.
5. Do not try to solve all the problems alone. Avoid conflicts that may occur by having a third party aid in the setting of limits and assignment of tasks, if the employee disagrees with the restricted assignment.
6. Do not allow talk of pain. Encourage normal, healthy behavior.
7. Steer the employees to professional help if they appear to need assistance as they re-adjust to working.
8. Recognize need and restrictions as real.

KINDS OF INJURIES SEEN AND RESULTS

The workers seen in the early years of the program had injuries that were many and varied. They included employees who could use only one hand, welders who ordinarily climbed on box cars to complete repairs who could no longer climb, men with lifting restrictions due to back strain, and those who needed bench-type sitting jobs for a period of time before being able to return to more mobile assignments. However, once the first few persons were successfully returned and cases were brought to completion, the program was 'off and running'.

In the first twelve months of the program 10,208 man hours were saved by developing temporary, restricted work assignments for 104 individuals. A savings of $127,408.00 in lost wages was realized. Over the years, as the program has expanded, this figure has increased four-fold. In addition, everyone involved has agreed that numerous re-injuries have been prevented by the gradual re-entry of injured workers to the work force. The program also successfully reduced lost time due to low back strain by 27 percent and lost time for all other injuries by 21 percent. In addition to the cost savings realized from the restricted work program, occupational therapy intervention in the rehabilitation and placement of severely injured employees requiring permanent accommodation saves an average of $1,509,000.00 per year in claim payout.

CASE STUDY

One case of a severely injured employee will be discussed in detail. In December of 1979, RP, a 32 year old railroad conductor fell, sustaining a bimalleolar fracture of the left ankle. He was initially treated with a closed reduction which proved unsuccessful. Eventually he had an open reduction and internal repair of the ankle. Severe ankle pain developed and in October of 1980 an evaluation by surgeons revealed marked loss of joint space with many bony changes in the distal tibia and talus. Therefore arthrodesis of the ankle was performed several months later. This resulted in an infected hematoma that required still further surgery and debridement. RP underwent final surgery for the removal of the internal fixation pins in May of 1981 and after rigorous therapy was discharged from medical care in September of 1981. He had now been not working for almost two years.

During RP's period of recuperation, the occupational therapist met with him frequently, serving as a coordinator for arranging medical care, therapy and vocational assessment. He was encouraged during that time to develop his interest in selling real estate, a job he could do while in a cast and on crutches. Arrangements were made to pay for a course he would need to be licensed to sell real estate and he was enrolled. This plan kept RP active and involved in the working community, which he enjoyed.

However, RP's first love was railroading and it was definitely more lucrative than real estate sales in a small town during rough economic times. He really wanted to return to his former job. At the time of his medical discharge he was restricted: from walking long distances or on uneven ground, from climbing and from lifting over 50 pounds. All of these activities are routine for a freight train conductor, his former job.

Vocational evaluation had shown that RP had better than average learning ability and good verbal and reasoning skills. Therefore, it was concluded that he would be able to pass the test for passenger conductor with minimal difficulty, and he did. With this test behind him, only one hurdle remained. The union had to be convinced that he be allowed to work, restricted to passenger service only, without affecting his seniority. After negotiation this was accomplished and RP returned to work in November of 1981 in his 'accommodated' position. He remains an employee today with an unblemished work record and good reports from all supervisors. If RP had not returned to gainful employment or had worked at a lesser paying job, the railroad could have had a claim payout equalling his wage loss of $35,000.00 per year to age 65. An additional award for 'pain and suffering' might have brought this figure to over a million dollars. Such is not an uncommon claim settlement in the railroad industry.

SUMMARY AND CONCLUSIONS

The story of how one occupational therapist developed and conducted a rehabilitation program in the railroad industry using occupational therapy philosophies and principles has been related. The results in concrete dollar savings as well as in the improved and safer function of workers in the industry were illustrated. A case example of a person with a typical worker injury was given. Both company and union officials, as well as employees themselves have been shown as interested and cooperative with such a preventive and rehabilitation program.

Mary Reilly was credited with the thought that "occupational therapy is directed toward enabling man to fulfill his innate need of occupation and the rich and varied stimuli that solving life problems provides him. Humans are occupational creatures who cannot be healthy in the absence of occupation."[6] Industrial rehabilitation is based on these concepts. These principles, that are the foundation of our profession, certainly support the need for and responsibility of the occupational therapist to carve a role in industrial medicine.

REFERENCES

1. Meyer, A: The philosophy of occupational therapy. Arch Occup Ther 1:1 10, 1922
2. Spackman, CS: Co-ordination of occupational therapy with other allied medical and related services. In Occupational Therapy, 3rd Ed., Philadelphia: Lippincott, p.1, 1963
3. Cromwell, F: Statement to the Joint Commission on Accreditation of Hospitals, Chicago, Illinois, June 10, 1972, Am J Occup Ther 26:3A-3B, 1972

4. The Role of the occupational therapist in vocational rehabilitation. A position paper, American Occupational Therapy Association, April 1980

5. Florence, DW: The Employee's reaction to a work related injury. Minneapolis, Mn: Sister Kenny Inst. (unpublished), 1980

6. Reilly, M: Occupational therapy can be one of the great ideas of twentieth century medicine. Am J Occup Ther 16:5, 1962

Work Center:
A School-Based Program
for Vocational Preparation of
Special Needs Children and Adolescents

Karen Jacobs, MS, OTR/L
Nancy Mazonson, MS, OTR/L
Kathy Pepicelli, OTR/L
Irene Clague, OTR/L
Wynne Leekoff, COTA/L

ABSTRACT. Changing one's role from student to worker is often a difficult transition today, especially when options for employment are linked with specialized training. For the handicapped adolescent it is almost impossible without very special training and guidance. Recent legislation affecting the handicapped mandated that efforts to assist this process shall begin two years prior to the student's graduation or at age twenty. Some writers insist that such supportive programming should begin when students are quite young and that it should be conducted within realistic 'work' environments.

Recognizing this need, the occupational therapy staff in a private school for special needs children and adolescents have taken a proactive stance and have initiated a work program for all students beginning as early as age 10. This paper describes the pilot Work Center, organized within a school and structured on a rehabilitation workshop model.

The Education of All Handicapped Children Act (Public Law 94-142) was enacted in 1975 and implemented beginning 1978. Many students now in programs funded under this legislation are

All five authors are occupational therapists employed at Little People's/Learning Prep School, West Newton, MA. Karen Jacobs is Director of Development, Nancy Mazonson, Director of Occupational Therapy, the other three staff therapists.

This article is dedicated to Elyse Mark.

This article appears jointly in *Work-Related Programs in Occupational Therapy* (The Haworth Press, 1985) and *Occupational Therapy in Health Care,* Volume 2, Number 4 (Winter 1985/1986).

47

reaching an age when vocational preparation should become a primary focus in their learning. Further, it is apparent that many handicapped youngsters have difficulty preparing for entry into the work world. Some writers indicate that work-related programming, started at a young age and reinforced in a 'work' environment can substantially assist students in acquiring the behaviors needed for them to become workers.[1] Common models of rehabilitation workshops can be integrated with programs in schools and thus more directly address work preparation needs. Work Center, a pilot program at The Little People's/Learning Prep School in West Newton, Massachusetts, has been designed to provide work preparation in a school setting, as well as assessment, training and employment services and referrals to employers in the community. This paper will describe the Center and its programs which are implemented by the occupational therapy staff using the facilities and resources of the school and its community.

REHABILITATION WORKSHOP MODELS

Various settings have been developed for the purpose of training disabled individuals to acquire work-related behaviors and skills. Rehabilitation workshops are one example. In the United States, such facilities are typically operated by private, nonprofit corporations and serve adults with either developmental or emotional disabilities.[2] Created in response to needs of these populations, rehabilitation workshops offer assessment, training, employment and other rehabilitative services in controlled and protected working environments. In addition, the settings allow for the individuals to work at their own capacity and receive corresponding remuneration.

There are four principal categories of rehabilitation work settings:

Transitional Workshops—These workshops are designed for persons with good potential for competitive employment. Placement is usually short term in nature and focused on competitive employment or re-employment using assorted transitional employment and vocational readjustment activities.

Sheltered Workshops—These settings provide, through various simple to complex job tasks, substantial employment for persons who appear unable to work in or have never had employment in the competitive marketplace. Sheltered workshops can be distinguished from transitional ones because the stay is long-term and generally for those whose productivity is below competitive levels. Most often, facilities designated as sheltered workshops offer a combination of sheltered and transitional programming.

Work Activity Centers (WAC)—WAC's offer programs for individuals who are not appropriate for sheltered placement but who could benefit from exposure to work-related tasks. Bergman (1977) notes that work activity centers "provide . . . individualized developmental services . . . (which) build coping skills and abilities, enhance decision-making processes, foster independent or semi-independent living and develop vocational skills and related behaviors."[4] In addition, the individual's capacity for productivity is virtually not emphasized.

Nearly half of all rehabilitation work settings are work activity centers. They are the fastest growing category of work program largely as a result of the trend of returning to their communities hospitalized persons who still need organized activities.[3]

WAC's offer diverse programs, with some engaging in crafts, while others concentrate on subcontract work. For many clients, this placement is an entry point to subsequent work-related programming.

Avocational or Day Adult Activity Center—The centers provide a day care environment serving as an alternative to institutionalization. Such centers are defined as "facilities with a developmental program of structured training for the most severely and profoundly impaired individuals who are unprepared to profit from the vocational orientation of a work activity center program."[3]

While functional levels of clients may differ markedly in the four program categories, the facilities are similar in that all offer a mechanism to measure individual growth and the ability to graduate to higher levels. The separate titles may in fact be arbitrary, reflecting personal choice of agencies. In fact all are often generically called sheltered workshops.

SCHOOL-BASED WORK SETTINGS

A workshop environment in a school can be an ideal milieu or modality for developing work-related behaviors and skills in children/adolescents. A realistic approximation of work in industry can be offered in a protected/controlled environment within the school's boundaries. Several writers feel it is crucial to initiate work-related programming for the special needs child at an early age. Such activity helps the child incorporate basic work attitudes and skills into a well-learned repertoire of behaviors. Often these behaviors are underdeveloped because of limited exposure (or lack of exposure) to the world of work, and limited career expectations by parents and society.[5] Activities which foster career awareness and afford exploration of vocational capabilities and interests should be introduced in a developmental manner. Lynch and colleagues note that, "training materials and work performance requirements should increasingly approximate actual industrial demands and training should move from the school to the actual work site as soon as possible."[1] Lynch further says, " . . . the classroom environment has little positive (and much negative) transfer value to the behaviors required in working environments, and, thus, the naturalistic environment should be tapped as quickly and as early as possible in the prevocational and vocational education of special needs youth."[1]

Justification for this type of programming comes from recent legislative action on a state level within Massachusetts. A newly enacted bill addresses the transitional planning needs of graduating students (or those who have reached 22) who have been receiving specialized schooling through Public Law 94-142. This legislation directs that programming begin two years prior to graduation or by age 20. Experience with handicapped young people has shown that the transition from student to worker roles is difficult and special services are needed. One response to both the Massachusetts legislation and the evident needs of the Learning Prep School population is The Work Center. The school and The Work Center will now be described.

LITTLE PEOPLE'S/LEARNING PREP SCHOOL (LPS)

The Little People's/Learning Prep School is a private, nonprofit day program offering services to a population of over 200 children/adolescents ranging in age from 6 to 22. Students have moderate to severe learning disabilities and/or exhibit a wide range of developmental delays. It is estimated nonetheless that approximately fifty percent of the students enrolled will be competitively employed following graduation. The other fifty percent will enter various types of rehabilitation workshops.

Occupational therapy services in the school address visual, perceptual-motor and work-related needs of the students. Careful observations of older adolescents making their first attempts to seek competitive employment have shown that basic work-related skills and behaviors were deficient. Students were having difficulty both getting and keeping jobs. The Occupational Therapy Department responded to these problems by initiating a pilot work program designed to introduce and develop work-related behaviors. Work Center evolved from this decision.

WORK CENTER

Based on a rehabilitation philosophy, Work Center has been designed to provide assessment, training, and employment activities as well as referral for job placement. Programming ranges from very basic activities that incorporate work-related behaviors and skills to actual work/study placement in the community (or in the school itself) in which students are paid accordingly to their levels of production. Sixty percent of the students in LPS are involved with the Center as a part of their program schedules. Typically students arrive at the Center, punch in on a time clock and then enter a self-contained room in which a rehabilitation workshop milieu is offered. Elements of this environment include therapists representing themselves as work supervisors, students interacting as co-workers, and routines that require clearly defined (and posted) rules of work conduct. The room itself is subdivided into work stations as well as break/lounge and personal hygiene areas. The remainder of this paper will describe the assessment activities used to identify trainees for Work Center and to place them in levels matching their needs.

ASSESSMENT

Students are referred to the Center by their teachers or therapists. Initially they are assessed by the occupational therapy staff to determine what services of the Center they need. Using adapted versions of the Prevocational Assessment and Curriculum Guide (PACG) staff are able to analyze work-related behaviors and skills. The PACG is an inventory which assesses behavior, interaction, self help skills considered necessary for successful entry into sheltered employment. The test has been subjected to validity and reliability studies and reflects contributions from rehabilitation workshops nationwide. The test further provides a rating scale defining levels of functioning necessary for entry to sheltered employment in nine behavior and skill areas. Accordingly if students are already functioning above sheltered levels they are not admitted to the Work Center.

The skill areas addressed by the PACG include behavior skills: attendance/endurance, independence, production, learning, behavior, and interaction skills: communication, social, grooming/eating and toileting skills.

An adapted version of the PACG is sometimes used. This adapted version is necessary to meet the needs of the younger population. The LPS staff feel that learning how to work is more important initially than focusing on production rates. Further, designing a shorter version of the test was essential with students having limited task focus. Most testing is administered to groups.

Based on these requirements a checklist for use with younger students was developed combining items from both the PACG and the Jacobs Prevocational Skills Assessment (JPSA). JPSA is composed of 15 tasks designed to assess performance in specific work-related skill areas.[5]

The resulting Work Center/Prevocational Occupational Therapy Inventory (POTI) essentially reflects the same categories of behavior and interaction skills as the standard PACG used with the older students.

Independence—the amount of supervision required to perform a structured task. Evidence of ability to do independent problem solving and decision making, to maintain an organized work area; and develop ways of doing things that compensate for fine motor, eye-hand and perceptual deficits PACG (7 items), POTI (10 items).

Production—the ability to perform tasks involving matching and sorting, to sequence steps of a task, the ability to monitor the quality of work, and to maintain or increase production levels PACG (8 items), POTI (12 items).

Learning—the ability to follow visual, verbal and/or written directions from simple to multi-step, tasks PACG (6 items) POTI (5 items).

Behavior—the ability to follow Work Center rules and deal with frustration appropriately PACG (8 items), POTI (6 items).

Structured Communication/Social Skills—the ability to communicate basic needs and to interact appropriately with co-workers and supervisor during the structured work periods PACG (5 items), POTI (6 items).

Unstructured Social Skills—the ability to interact with others appropriately during an informal break PACG (2 items), POTI (7 items).

Work Center students functioning at obviously higher levels who are referred for evaluation are assessed using the regular PACG, modified only with respect to the work environment items. Any of these students whose performance falls below entry level for sheltered employment in two or more skills areas are referred to the Center for remediation services. Those whose performance is at or above entry level are referred directly to LPS vocational placement personnel. All students tested whose scores indicate need for Work Center programs, are assigned to levels of training according to testing results. Those levels will now be described.

WORK CENTER TRAINING LEVELS

Upon completion of a Work Center/Prevocational Occupational Therapy Inventory or PACG, and based on scoring, students are assigned to one of four levels (A-D) to indicate the kind of programming recommended. A is the lowest level of functioning, D the highest. Levels are characterized by staff to student ratios, length of training sessions, skills and behaviors to be addressed and complexity of tasks involved. Training at all levels is conducted under supervision of occupational therapy staff, who are also responsible for regular re-evaluation as well as reporting of student progress. The amount and nature of Center involvement is determined on an individual basis depending on the student's level of functioning and long term goals. As a result, programming can provide services which incorporate elements of all four types of rehabilitation workshops described earlier. Movement from one level to the next is based on informal assessment of the students' abilities to manage the staff ratio, length of session and performance demands of the next level.[6]

Level A—Programming at this level has a staff to student ratio ranging from 1:2 to 1:4. Sessions are for 30 minutes without a formal break period and include assignment to two tasks. Focus at this level is on the introduction of training in work-related behaviors, e.g., independent transit, working without disruption, communicating basic needs appropriately. Tasks assigned require following one step multi-modal directions and doing simple matching/sorting activities. Basic functions requiring fine motor and eye-hand coordination, visual discrimination and perceptual skills are also incorporated into tasks. Simulated 'jobs' used include sorting objects by one variable (e.g., color, size or shape) and simple packaging.

Level B—This level operates with the same staff to student ratio as level A (1:2 to 1:4) but length of sessions is extended to 45 minutes with a 5 to 10 minute break. Program focus is on the refinement and reinforcement of previously established work-related behaviors and the development of skills necessary to complete additional simulated workshop 'jobs'. Tasks involve being able to sort by one and two variables, and require organizational skills, basic decision making and the ability to attend, follow and sequence 2/3 step verbal and visual directions. Basic functions mentioned in level A are also incorporated into tasks by choices of sizes, of complexity of materials handling, speed of process. Common terminology associated with working, e.g., quality control, inventory control, is introduced. The break is introduced to present opportunity for staff to observe informal socialization skills and use of unstructured time. Simulated 'jobs' include collating, packaging and sorting by at least two variables such as shape and color, and doing all the steps involved in packaging of various kinds.

Level C—The staff to student ratio at this level is 1:4 or 1:5. Length of sessions ranges from 45-60 minutes, and sessions include a 10 minute break. Training focus is on activities that afford maintenance of now established work-related behaviors and skills with the addition of opportunity for increasing independence of function and decision-making, completing a task by following a model or sample, following 3 or more visual, verbal and/or written directions and increasing production rate and accuracy. Students are encouraged to recognize and apply ways to compensate for any deficits in fine motor function, eye-hand coordination and perceptual function. Simulated 'jobs' include sorting by 2 or more variables, packaging of multi-item materials, doing tasks typical of office work and engaging in simple assembly activities.

Level D—The assignment to this level is limited to students who have completed successfully all the activities of Level C and are at least 16 years old. Most of the jobs at this level are secured through subcontracts from nearby community businesses and students are paid for their production. The staff to student ratio can be from 1:5 to 1:12 and work sessions are 50 to 100 minutes long at present, with one 10 minute break. Future scheduling will extend work time and gradually build toward regular half-day work periods.

At this level of training, students are expected to be able to refine and add to behaviors and skills established at level C. Emphasis is placed on increasing speed of production while maintaining consistent quality. Workers each chart their own daily production and receive supervision designed to facilitate further understanding of issues related to work speed, quality and pay. Jobs in subcontract work which have been secured have included various kinds of simple to complex operations, involving assembly, packaging, bulk mailing and collating. (See Figure 1.)

REFERRAL

All students who have reached Level D are monitored by the school's vocational placement coordinator. Students whose performance in seven or more skill categories meets or exceeds entry level standards for sheltered work are referred for possible work/study placement. In addition, students who are approaching graduation within 1-2 years are considered ready for work/study placement.

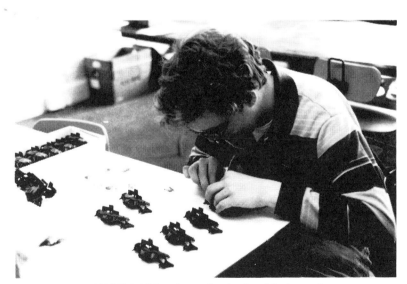

FIGURE 1. LPS student performing Level D piecework

Jobs can be in volunteer, sheltered, or competitive settings. Participation in the Center ends when students are placed in work/study jobs.

CONTRACT PROCUREMENT

Obtaining subcontracts of suitable work tasks is an ongoing demand accomplished by continually locating job possibilities thru both formal and informal contacts. Formal sources include printed directories (yellow pages and local business listings) to contact companies which might have subcontract work needs; contacting social and health and welfare organizations (other workshops, non-profit organizations); and advertising services available at LPS in local newspapers. From one formal contact, an arrangement was established with a large local sheltered workshop which needed subcontract help. During their periods of contract overload, this workshop provides numerous jobs for which LPS students receive piecework pay.

Informal job sources are those that occur from professional and personal contacts of staff. For example, the Center now does the collating and bulk mailing for the Massachusetts Association for Occupational Therapy.

CONCLUSION

Initial results from the first year of the Work Center pilot program have been favorable. This program, seen by staff as proactive, has resulted in students being able to translate their acquired work-related behaviors and skills to classroom activities and into vocational workshops (another aspect of the LPS services). It is hoped that this ability to generalize their skills will continue as students are placed in assignments requiring higher level work functions, e.g., work/study offerings at LPS or in community-based sheltered or regular employment. Since measures of relative achievement in each level are still crude, staff hope they can devise an instrument to measure student progress in concrete, employer-focused terms and to serve as a means by which selection of placements for jobs within the school and community can be better done.

Parents and community friends of LPS programs see the addition of a program such as Work Center as an important building block in helping special needs students move to roles as workers. It appears that LPS can indeed assist this vital transition.

REFERENCES

1. Lynch KP, Kiernan WE, Stark JA (Eds): *Prevocational and Vocational Education for Special Needs Youth: a Blueprint for the 1980's.* Baltimore: Paul H. Brookes Publishing Co., 1982

2. Demor, Z: *Directory of Sheltered Workshops.* Information and referral. United Way of Massachusetts Bay, 87 Kilby Street, Boston, MA 02109, 1983

3. Wright, GN: *Total Rehabilitation,* Boston: Little, Brown and Co., 1980

4. Bergmen, A: A guide to establishing an activity center for mentally retarded persons. Washington, D.C.: President's committee on employment of the handicapped, 1977

5. Jacobs, K: *Occupational Therapy: Work-related Programs and Assessments,* Boston: Little, Brown and Co., 1985

6. Mithaug, DE, Mar, DK and Stewart, JE: *Prevocational Assessment and Curriculum Guide.* Washington: Exceptional Education. 1978

A Private Practice Work Evaluation Unit

Thelma Wellerson Hook, MA, OTR, ASHT

ABSTRACT. A private practice, free standing work evaluation center was established in November 1982 to serve a large metropolitan area in northern California. Originally conceived to evaluate and treat persons with traumatic hand and/or upper extremity injuries, the practice has now expanded to include services for industrially injured workers, persons with personal injury claims who have sustained a broad range of physical and/or emotional disabilities, as well as individuals receiving State rehabilitation services.

The role of the occupational therapist within this vocationally oriented unit is varied and has proven highly beneficial for individuals with various kinds of disabilities. While occupational therapists have moved in and out of this area of practice over the years, they now seem to be re-establishing themselves as viable and significant parts of work-related programming. Their unique skills and broad expertise enhance overall care of impaired workers and 'bridge the gap' between medical and vocational services.

This paper presents a brief description of programming in a work unit and concludes with recommendations for others interested in this area of practice.

Occupational therapists are well suited to be 'the bridge' between the medical and vocational phases of the rehabilitation process for persons having disability from injury or illness. During the last two years there has been a ground swell of attention by therapists in offering vocational services. This rediscovery has been demonstrated by increases in the numbers of professional articles, textbooks, conferences, workshops and informal meetings appearing, as well as a growth in networking of therapists involved in offering work related services.

Thelma Wellerson Hook, an active member of The American Society of Hand Therapists, is Director and Owner of Hand Therapy and Rehabilitation Associates, Inc. and Hook Associates, *The WorkSolution,* 251 E. Hacienda Suite A, Campbell, CA 95008.

This article appears jointly in *Work-Related Programs in Occupational Therapy* (The Haworth Press, 1985) and *Occupational Therapy in Health Care,* Volume 2, Number 4 (Winter 1985/1986).

In addition to these visible manifestations of the rediscovery of this area of practice, the nation's economy has presented therapists working within the medical model some hard facts that also have stimulated exploration of other areas of practice. Health costs nationally are rising drastically. With the efforts in cost containment have come many cutbacks affecting occupational therapists: layoffs, shrinkage of perimeters of practice, consolidation of departments, as well as the federal limitations on reimbursement for services. Because all these moves directly or indirectly affect sources of referrals and revenue for occupational therapy, many therapists have concluded that the time has come to seek and serve referrals outside the medical model. One of these options is by developing services based on the profession's traditional role in vocational evaluation and training.

This paper will describe one therapist's experience in developing just such a practice and will conclude with recommendations which might be helpful to others thinking of work-related programming.

INCEPTION OF THE WORKSOLUTION

Hand Therapy and Rehabilitation Associates, Inc. was founded in 1976 in Los Gatos, California. It was established as a private practice, medically oriented center offering hand therapy services to patients of private, industrial and hospital-based physicians in northern California. The sole purpose of this medically prescribed treatment program is to treat industrial and private patients with traumatic hand and upper extremity injuries and dysfunctions. Each member of the multi-professional staff in the center is committed to return the patient to his own occupation as quickly as possible and as soon as medically feasible.

As an adjunct to what has proven to be a highly successful hand therapy office, *The WorkSolution* was established as a free-standing and separate evaluation unit in November 1982. *The WorkSolution* is therefore a private practice, *non-medically oriented* office located in an urban area in the midst of the high tech industry of Santa Clara Valley in California. Philosophically it was seen as important that *The WorkSolution* be a free standing office to differentiate the individual served from the role of 'patient' in the medical rehabilitation process to the role of 'client' in the vocational rehabilitation process.

Clients seen are referred still by medical sources, but also more often by insurance claim coordinators, private rehabilitation specialists or employers themselves who are eager to have employees return to their jobs. Types of injuries seen are widely diverse, characteristic of the kinds of industry surrounding the center, and include both upper and lower extremity injuries as well as back problems and persons with chronic pain from whatever disabling source.

All staff in the center have special training in the activities they perform, be it interviewing and administering various interest and ability tests, or counseling regarding return to work with or without job modification, or the actual work activities used to provide work simulation, work hardening, or general conditioning. Occupational therapists are either certified work evaluators or certified work adjustment specialists.

SERVICES OFFERED

The WorkSolution now offers the following programs and services.

Work Capacity Evaluation (WCE): This involves an extensive and individualized assessment program with clients participating in a six hour day of various activities for a minimum of five to a maximum of ten days. Supervision of activity is one therapist to four clients. The evaluation process includes a comprehensive assessment of the individual's aptitudes, interests, physical tolerances, temperament, attitudes and work skills. Persons are referred for WCE to determine work potential and needs for alteration of or change in occupation.

Numerous modalities are utilized by staff in conducting this assessment. These include aptitude tests, interest inventories, dexterity tests, and performance on various work samples such as from the Valpar, Singer, W.E.S.T and TOWER systems. The ultimate results of the work capacity evaluation can provide the referring agent with specific information about abilities helpful for developing realistic rehabilitation plans for the injured worker. Information obtained from this testing is obviously extensive and becomes also extremely beneficial in pointing to new directions when a career change is required due to an industrial injury.

Work Tolerance Screening: Often injured workers simply need opportunity to build up tolerance for work after lengthy periods of layoff. Thus this program is designed to offer a structured environment in which that can occur. The screening therefore is a very specific and intensive program offering activity for a minimum of three hours to a maximum of seven hours a day over a three day span. Supervision is one to one in order to clearly establish the present physical abilities of the injured worker. The screening includes standard tests of range of motion, muscle strength, grip and pinch strength, sensation, dexterity, tolerance to vibration and/or hot and cold, ability to lift under load and carry, and ability to apply torque with small and large tools. Activities are undertaken and designed to address the particular disability of the client. In addition, there is an appraisal of the client's physical ability to perform specific work-related activities utilizing work samples in controlled and supervised settings, again with attention to both testing and accommodating the specific limitations of the client.

The results of work tolerance screening provide the referring agent a baseline of specific abilities which aid him in establishing realistic work goals and job alternatives with and for the injured worker.

Work Hardening: There are two types of work hardening offered, medical work hardening, and vocational work hardening. *Medical work hardening* is used to facilitate returning the injured worker to his usual and customary job or for aiding in the determination of 'Qualified Injured Worker' status. *Vocational work hardening* is used with an individual already determined to be a 'qualified injured worker' prior to his (a) on-the-job training, (b) entry into a vocational training program, or (c) direct job placement.

In either case this is a progressive individualized physical conditioning and training program in which the client is involved in activities during a period of three weeks, beginning with two hours a day the first week, four hours the second week, and six hours daily the third week. Modifications to this time schedule can be made when deemed appropriate by the evaluator upon notification of the referring agent.

Modalities used are specific work tasks and activities such as soldering, building maintenance activities, and mechanical drafting. In addition to planning work for stamina and productivity, the evaluator monitors client attendance, consistency of performance, temperament, concentration, memory, quality of interpersonal relationships, ability to handle supervision, general work attitudes along with other specific job related behaviors. The planning of the work hardening program is aimed ultimately toward increasing the client's general physical and emotional stamina so as to be able to meet the demands of either part or full time employment in his specific skill area.

Job Analysis: The purpose of this part of the center's program is to help match client ability with job by carefully analyzing the requirements of the employment setting and operation. Knowing job requirements helps to guide work hardening as well as to see adaptations of work procedures if necessary. Performed on site in industry the service assesses both physical and environmental demands of a specific job setting. The analysis, therefore, provides the referral agent with a realistic, first hand picture of actual job duties that an injured worker would have to be able to do to return to work.

The analyst notes in detail all the job skills that are required of the injured worker so as to match demands with disability as well as assets. Such a careful look at jobs often uncovers potentials not realized by either client or employer. Detailed reports and recommendations of the site visit are submitted to the referring agent.

On-the-Job Assessment: Closely related to job analysis is on-the-job assessment in which an intensive one-to-one service is offered in which the therapist evaluates the injured worker's endurance, tolerance to pain and actual performance *in a specific job setting.* The purpose of this service is to observe the client at work, to analyze his physical ability to perform those tasks necessary for the job within the framework of industrial performance standards, and to consider performance alternatives if there are problems. The results of this assessment include recommendations that may involve one of the following: (a) return to the job as it exists (no change in job), (b) modification of the individual's way of doing his work, the work processes themselves or aspects of the job site, or (c) seek alternative job placement.

Job Site Modification or Worker 'Modification': A natural accompaniment of on the job assessment is a search for ways of making job performance possible. Thus the therapist offers a service in which she analyzes the client, the job, and the place of work with an eye toward finding alternative solutions to how a job can be done within the framework of industrial performance standards. Results of such additional analysis suggest recommendations such as including the application of ergonomic principles for job site modifications (e.g., raising a chair), or fabrication of adaptive equipment designed especially to enable an individual client to do a task (e.g., a thumb splint), instruction in compensatory body mechanics that the client can learn or unlearn in order to safely perform his job (e.g., use of shoulder motion instead of hand to do an action, or training the worker to do certain things with the other hand), or modification of job skills and equipment (e.g., use of a special portable desoldering tool that requires one hand operation vs. a traditional desoldering tool that requires two hand control, or providing built-up knobs, handles, switches that will enable the client to do his work and still meet industrial standards.

Job Search Skills Training: Many clients who must change jobs or who have not worked for a long time (or ever) need assistance in finding suitable jobs and applying for them successfully. Accordingly, the center offers job search skills training in which a two week program is offered on a daily basis covering a minimum of four hours a day. Clients are grouped with one trainer for up to six clients. The program offers information and training on how to use a telephone, write effective resumes, how to present oneself at interviews and fill out applications. In addition, clients are given material support from the unit including access to telephones for calling employers as well as secretarial support, stationery, postage for letters of inquiry and/or application. The program also is structured so as to provide daily motivation and social support to the unemployed individual. The goal of this program is to fill jobs and reduce unemployment of industrially injured workers by offering personalized support during difficult transitions.

Corporate Consultation: A final service offered is to industries themselves in which consultation is available to focus on problems of safety, injury, efficiency of workers. Therapists consult in all areas of a company's activities as requested either on a single visit or long term basis. The specific skills offered in this service are related to prevention of hand and upper extremity injury to employees, as well as for application of general principles of ergonomics and body mechanics to job functions.

Results of such intervention and corrective actions can reduce corporate costs significantly and have been well received.

SUMMARY

In summary, this paper has described a particular way one occupational therapist is involved in work-related programming. The particular program came about because of a belief that the occupational therapist has not only traditionally been a part of vocational activities, but also because of having special knowledge and abilities to 'bridge the gap' of patients' needs between the medical and vocational rehabilitation programs is a logical one to carry out such activities.

It was shown that the need for such work-focused services is growing because of the constant changes in health care delivery and expansion of the potential marketing areas due to changes in reimbursement practices for occupational therapy. It was also stated that *The WorkSolution* has proven to be a viable and successful program in which occupational therapists serve as vocational evaluators and work adjustment specialists. Specific aspects of the service were described.

CONCLUSION

Offering work-related services for persons with disability from injury or illness is a growing opportunity for occupational therapists. The needs are there. Despite active safety programs in industry, many workers are injured on the job each year. It is dollar-wise for management and insurance companies to seek ways to return workers to employment as soon as possible. *The WorkSolution* and other occupational therapy programs like it can provide the services needed to achieve this goal.

The Occupational Therapist's Role in Employee Health Promotion Programs

Annette Mungai, MS, OTR

ABSTRACT. The first challenge in developing an effective health promotion program for employees is the performance of a health needs assessment on the target population. In an effort to meet this challenge, 600 corporate employees were surveyed and compared with respect to the allotment of time to work, leisure, and self/family care activities; health risk factors; perceived health; and activity satisfaction. The results of the study indicated that the employees participating in the corporate health and fitness programs were not the high risk individuals who consume the majority of the corporate medical dollar.

The role of the occupational therapist in meeting the needs of high risk employees is discussed. A brief review of the literature addresses research efforts in the area of health promotion in industry and the role of the occupational therapist in disease prevention. The appropriateness of occupational therapy education, training and theory in relation to health promotion programs and the utilization of the five occupational performance components in the evaluation of employee populations is outlined.

Finally, the role of the occupational therapist working in specific areas of health promotion is reviewed, including: back pain reduction, substance abuse treatment, cardiac fitness/rehabilitation and hypertension control, smoking cessation, weight reduction, stress management, industrial accident and injury prevention, and self-responsibility for health instruction.

In 1982, the nation's medical bill was 322 billion dollars, 10.5 percent of the gross national product.[1] It has been determined that

Annette Mungai is a registered occupational therapist at Ralph K. Davies Medical Center, Castro and Duboce Streets, San Francisco, CA 94114.

The author would like to thank Karen Diasio, MA, OTR, FAOTA; Lela Llorens, PhD, OTR, FAOTA; Patsy Harmon; and ESL Incorporated for their assistance and support in the completion of this study. This research was conducted in partial fulfillment of the requirements for a Master of Science degree at San Jose State University.

This article appears jointly in *Work-Related Programs in Occupational Therapy* (The Haworth Press, 1985) and *Occupational Therapy in Health Care,* Volume 2, Number 4 (Winter 1985/1986).

67

53 percent of premature deaths in the United States are related to lifestyle behavior, yet less than 2.5 percent of the total health care expenditure has been devoted to prevention.[1,2] Additionally, an estimated 8 percent to 9 percent of the gross national product is attributable to the indirect costs of health care, such as losses in productivity associated with poor employee health.[1] Business and industry are paying 40 percent of health care costs in the United States.[3] With medical expenses rising at a rate of 10 percent per year, industries are looking for alternative methods of keeping employees healthy and thereby reducing health care costs.

A variety of professionals and non-professionals are defining roles for themselves in the expanding arena of health care in industry. Health promotion in business and industry involves the initial indentification of employee health risk factors, which have a strong correlation with lifestyle induced illnesses; followed by the implementation of programs to reduce risk factors, thereby improving employee health, increasing productivity, reducing absenteeism, and ultimately reducing corporate health care costs. Health promotion programs focusing on the occupational performance areas of work, leisure, and self-care are considered to be appropriate for business and industrial settings. This approach to intervention incorporates the occupational performance components of sensory integration, neuromuscular function, cognitive function, psychological function, and social interaction.[4,5]

Before an occupational therapy theory-based health promotion program can be appropriately implemented in business and industry, the needs of the employee population must be determined with respect to lifestyle behaviors. The purpose of this research was to assess the health care needs of a corporate population by focusing on the balance of work, leisure, and self/family care and by determining the presence or absence of health risk factors within the employee lifestyle. This is a first step in the development of the role of occupational therapy in the field of health promotion in business and industry.

LITERATURE REVIEW

Four central bodies of literature pertain to this research. These are: occupational therapy literature, time management literature, health and medical literature, and business literature.

Limited occupational therapy literature exists on the role of occupational therapists in primary and secondary prevention through health promotion. However, a number of articles which discuss the concept of balance in work, leisure, and self-care activities present the theoretical base upon which this study was conducted. Reilly stated that occupational therapy's base is to be found in the understanding of human organization as a balance between work, play, rest and sleep.[6] Clark presented the idea of a flexible balance of work, play and self-maintenance activities as a means by which people maintain health.[7]

Shannon also studied work-play activities, and suggested that an individual's daily living activities generally consisted of work and time free from work. Shannon did not recommend equality in the hours devoted to work and play but proposed that there must be in every individual's life opportunities for work, for rest, and for play, proportional to each individual's needs. Finally, Shannon suggested that deficits in work-play experiences can contribute to dysfunction and result in a proneness to maladaptation.[8]

Studies reviewed in the time management literature focused primarily on the allocation of time to various activities within a given period.[9,10,11] This topic has not been studied with respect to the impact of time allotment on an individual's health and activity satisfaction.

The health education and medical literature relevant to this study were focused on the transformation of medicine from a technology based, curative approach to a more human based prevention orientation. A topic of importance in this area is the collection of data that directly tests and documents the effects of industrial health promotion in the treatment and prevention of physical and mental illness.[12,13]

Cox and Shepard studied employees of two large Canadian life insurance companies over time to determine the effects of an employee fitness program on job satisfaction and absenteeism. Employee fitness program participants demonstrated: decreased absenteeism, increased work performance, more positive attitudes towards work, and decreased stress and tension.[12] Many industries have made the first steps towards health promotion through the implementation of fitness and exercise programs for a number of reasons. The greatest impetus for considering exercise as a health modality is its potential role in the prevention of heart disease and its use in rehabilitation.[14,15,16,17,18,19,20]

Physical fitness, while important, is only one of the many areas that contribute to higher levels of wellness. Cost benefit studies of multifaceted health promotion programs are not easily conducted due to difficulty in assigning monetary values to health outcomes and attributing specific benefits to specific programs. In addition, significant changes in group health status brought about by health promotion programs do not surface for at least three to five years.[21]

Although statistical documentation of financial benefits of health promotion programs in business and industry is still incomplete, this is the principle topic of question and study with which business literature preoccupies itself. Over the past twenty-five years, the scope of employee benefits has expanded significantly and cost has increased far faster than wages. While wages have increased 98 percent over the 10 year period from 1967-1977, health insurance benefits increased in cost by 284 percent.[22]

The most extensive research related to the cost-effective utilization of health promotion programs in business has been conducted in the U.S.S.R. Pravosudov, of the Iesgaft State Institute of Physical Culture in Leningrad, conducted a study on the effect of physical exercise on health and economic efficiency. The Leningrad study reported that: (a) workers taking part in fitness activity missed fewer days due to respiratory and non-respiratory diseases; (b) the duration of sickness of individuals involved with fitness was significantly less than that of the sedentary counterparts; (c) persons taking part in fitness activity consulted doctors four times less than those not engaged in physical training; (d) unfit workers were two to three times more vulnerable to industrial accidents than their active colleagues; (e) workers who were fit had a higher working capacity—depending on the task, their output was between two to five percent higher.[23,2]

The concepts of disease prevention and health promotion in industry have expanded rapidly in recent years. Often there is a tendency to discuss the issues in non-analytical terms. Aside from the sensationalistic approach, efforts are being made to carefully study the issues related to health promotion in industry and to the role of the occupational therapist in disease prevention.

DETAILS OF THE STUDY

The first challenge in developing an effective health promotion program for employees is the performance of a health needs assessment on the target population. The objectives of this study were to conduct such a needs assessment by evaluating the occupational behavior management skills of ESL Incorporated employees from an occupational therapy frame of reference and determining the presence or absence of health risk factors within the employees' lifestyle.

ESL Incorporated is located in Sunnyvale, California and is involved in communications research. ESL Incorporated has available for all employees an on-site fitness facility featuring a full line of Nautilus weight equipment, lifestyle stationary bicycles, an aerobic exercise room, limited free weights, a parcourse, a quarter mile jogging track, a basketball court, a sand volleyball court, horseshoe pits, and shower and locker facilities. In addition, noon-time health education classes are offered on smoking cessation, back care, medical self-help, blood pressure screening, weight control, nutrition, and fitness.

A systemic sampling technique was utilized to select 300 fitness program participants and 300 fitness program non-participants to be surveyed and compared with respect to the allotment of time to work, leisure, and self/family care activities; five health risk factors including blood pressure, years of tobacco smoking, quantity of tobacco smoked, caffeinated beverages consumed, and alcoholic beverages consumed; perceived health; and activity satisfaction.

The survey tool was a two-page self-administered questionnaire entitled, "Activity Patterns and Health Questionnaire". The first section of the questionnaire covered demographic variables in a checklist format (sex, age, highest educational level achieved, present job classification, full-time or part-time employment, sedentary or non-sedentary worker, and number of individuals cared for.

The second section included the researcher's definitions of work, leisure, and self/family care activities, each followed respectively by a question regarding the amount of time (hours and minutes) during an average workday the subject spent in work, leisure, and self/family care activities.

Section three presented health risk factors in a checklist format including: blood pressure, years of tobacco smoking, quantity of tobacco smoked, caffeinated beverages consumed, and alcoholic beverages consumed.

The final section covering perceived health and activity satisfaction included: a listing of the three leisure activities in which the subject was most likely to participate, a Cantril ladder for measuring the subject's level of perceived health, a Likert scale for reporting degree of satisfaction with the balance of activities in one's life, and finally, the opportunity to report the activity areas the individual would most want to change or improve.

Of the 600 questionnaires distributed, 249 were returned for a 41.5 percent return rate. One hundred and fifty-two (61 percent) were received from Group I consisting of fitness program participants, and 97 (39 percent) were received from Group II consisting of fitness program non-participants. The information obtained via the questionnaire was analyzed using the Statistical Package for the Social Sciences, second edition.[24]

Discriminant variable analysis was conducted and the following characteristics were found to distinguish Group I, fitness program participants: male, younger, better educated, more sedentary at work, responsible for fewer individuals in their personal life, work slightly more hours, spend slightly less time in the pursuit of leisure activities, spend slightly less time in self/family care, spend more time sleeping, not have high blood pressure, smoke less, drink fewer caffeinated beverages, drink slightly more alcohol, perform more active leisure activities, have a higher personal rating of perceived health, and indicate greater satisfaction with the balance of activities in one's life.

The following seven variables were found to statistically significantly differentiate between the two employee groups: age, highest educational level attained, number of individuals cared for, presence of high blood pressure, years of tobacco smoking, number of caffeinated beverages consumed, and number of sedentary leisure activities. Of these seven variables, five proved to be statistically significant in outlining a profile of the characteristics of employees who participate in corporate fitness programs. These employees tend to be: younger, more educated, non-smokers, participants in more active leisure activities, and demonstrative of greater satisfaction with the balance of activities in one's life.

The conclusions drawn from this study were:

1. The balance of work, leisure, and self/family care activities was similar for ESL Incorporated employees who participated in a corporate fitness program and for those employees who did not participate in a corporate fitness program.
2. ESL Incorporated employees who participated in a corporate fitness program differed significantly from those employees who did not participate in a corporate fitness program with respect to four out of five health risk factors evaluated.
3. Over 40 percent of all ESL Incorporated employees who responded to the questionnaire were undecided, dissatisfied, or

very dissatisfied with respect to the balance of activities in their lives.

4. The five research variables which were statistically significant in differentiating ESL Incorporated employees who participated in a corporate fitness program from those employees who did not participate in a corporate fitness program were: age, highest educational level attained, number of cigarettes, cigars, or pipes full of tobacco smoked, active leisure activities, and satisfaction with activity balance.

IMPLICATIONS FOR OCCUPATIONAL THERAPY

The results of this study indicate that the employees participating in the health and fitness program are those with fewer health risk factors, those who are the least likely to consume the corporate medical dollar. According to Pelletier, within any organization there is a small percentage of employees, usually 10 percent to 15 percent who utilize between 80 percent and 90 percent of all medical services paid for by the institution. [26] It is the costly rehabilitation and medical care of that small high risk percentage which could be reduced through the use of an occupational therapist in early detection and management of health risks, improving work conditions, and health education.

An occupational therapist's medical knowledge, in conjunction with her/his training in human behavior, activity analysis, and mind/body/environment interaction, produces a health professional with an excellent background for providing the services of health risk detection, work environment assessment and adaptation, and health education. An occupational therapist would augment an employee fitness program which focuses primarily on physical exercise. She/he would provide health promotion services appropriate for the high risk employee population, many of whom may be intimidated by or uninterested in a high performance physical fitness program.

The motivation and time management issues inherent to the process of lifestyle change and health enhancement indicate the appropriateness of a health promotion program based on an occupational therapy frame of reference. The occupational therapist would focus on the interaction of mind, body, and environment in the coordination and performance of work, leisure, and self-care activities. By analyzing activities, individuals or groups within a corporation could be led through a systematic and structured process to examine their daily routines, delete unnecessary activities, consider new options through creative problem solving, and reexamine priorities, thereby generally improving the quality of their lives and presumably the productivity of the corporation.[25]

Within the development of health enhancement programs in a hospital setting, the occupational therapist's efforts could be directed towards hospital employees and/or marketed to corporations. The hospital setting offers a unique compliment of health related personnel and equipment which could be incorporated into a wellness program, as well as an in-house population of employees to be used in the evaluation of a program's effectiveness before marketing to an outside corporation.

OCCUPATIONAL THERAPY APPROACHES

The occupational therapist would utilize activity performance within the areas of work, leisure, and self/family care as a basis for evaluation and intervention; with the inherent qualities of activity assessed through the five performance components of sensory integration, neuromuscular function, cognitive function, psychological function, and social interaction.[4,5]

Using the framework of the five occupational performance components there are a number of evaluations performed by an occupational therapist which would be appropriate for an employee population. With respect to neuromuscular function, the occupational therapist would evaluate: range of motion, muscular strength, flexibility, posture, endurance, body composition, and reaction time. Sensory integration evaluations would be appropriate for employees afflicted by alcohol and substance abuse. With respect to cognitive function, the occupational therapist would provide evaluation of employees' cognitive work skills and abilities, as well as work efficiency through work sample testing. With respect to psychological functioning, the occupational therapist would evaluate stress management, time management, work, leisure, and self-care activity balance, and pre-retirement planning. The occupational therapist would also utilize specific psychological evaluation tools appropriate for a corporate population such as the Personality Inventory, the Interest Checklist, and the Life Satisfaction Inventory. With respect to social functioning, the occupational therapist would utilize interviews and observation to assess interpersonal skills which may be interfering in the work place and at home.

Other evaluation services would include: evaluation of environmental health and safety, evaluation of work place accessibility for the disabled, comprehensive health risk appraisals, back injury, and other industrial injury evaluations.

SOME TARGET POPULATIONS

Within an employee health promotion program, the occupational therapist could work effectively in a number of areas incuding: back pain reduction, substance abuse treatment, cardiac fitness/rehabilitation and hypertension control, smoking cessation, weight reduction, stress management, industrial accident and injury prevention, and self-responsibility for health instruction.

In the instruction of *back pain* reduction classes, the occupational therapist woud educate the employee on pertinent back anatomy and physiology, instruct in the use of proper body mechanics during bending, reaching, carrying, and lifting activities, conduct task analysis for job as well as home tasks, make recommendations as to appropriate environmental adaptations such as proper chair and table heights, and utilize biofeedback when appropriate.

In the treatment of *substance abuse,* the occupational therapist would incorporate behavior modification with educational programs. Thorough assessment of work and home activity patterns in relation to alcohol/drug consumption would be conducted. The employee would be instructed on how to change lifestyle patterns which foster substance dependency and referred as necessary to substance abuse programs which support and facilitate efforts to terminate alcohol/drug addictions.

A *cardiac fitness*/rehabilitation and hypertension control program directed by an occupational therapist would include an evaluation of the employee's lifestyle patterns as well as a series of work capacity and home task evaluations. These evaluations would: identify the physical stresses of the employee's living situation, determine primary roles of the employee, analyze habit patterns and customary daily activities, and outline the employee's use of time. Intervention components of an occupational therapy based cardiac rehabilitation program would include: instruction on coronary artery disease and its effect on the heart, education in and reinforcement of lifestyle changes to facilitate risk factor management, instruction and training in activity modification and task self-monitoring to encourage a balance of activity and rest to facilitate recognition and avoidance of sudden stresses on the cardiovascular system, relaxation training to reduce stress on the cardiovascular system due to excess muscle tension, instruction in life goals management to facilitate transitions to vocational and leisure activities more suited to cardiac tolerance, and instruction in menu planning and cooking for a restricted diet.[27]

Within a *smoking cessation* program, the occupational therapist would provide instruction in behavior modification techniques to decrease smoking behavior, in conjunction with increasing employee's awareness of the direct impact of lifestyle patterns and activities on smoking. Peer support groups would also be utilized to provide an opportunity for discussion and support as the reduction in smoking begins to challenge other life habits and activities. In a *weight reduction* program, the occupational therapist would also utilize behavior modification and peer/family support as well as assist with nutrition instruction.

Stress management classes led by an occupational therapist would utilize relaxation techniques, increase self-awareness, mind-body control, and biofeedback. The incorporation of stress reduction techniques within the employee's average daily activity routine would be an integral part of the stress reduction program.

The role of the occupational therapist in industrial *accident and injury prevention* would include an evaluation of the work site followed by a series of recommendations for environmental modifications and adaptations, such as changing the height of work surfaces, modifying lighting systems, or providing additional support to the body in a specific work position.

Self-responsibility for health classes led by an occupational therapist would incorporate motivational techniques to encourage participation in and continued performance of activities for which the employee may not be intrinsically motivated but which are beneficial for health.

SUMMARY

The opportunities for an occupational therapist in employee health promotion are numerous, but before they can be fully realized, the philosophy and treatment techniques of occupational therapy must expand from a rehabilitation orientation working with the disabled to one that includes the prevention of disease and dysfunction and the promotion of health.

REFERENCES

1. Carr EM: Project results from two client settings. In the *Beyond Our Boundaries Presenter's Papers Organizational Development Network National Conference* Program, 1983, p. 224

2. Jacobs DT: *Getting Your Executives Fit.* Mountain View, CA: Anderson World, 1981

3. Deane B: Wellness in the workplace. *California Living Magazine,* 8, Oct. 10, 1982

4. AOTA: *Occupational Therapy Product Output Reporting System and Uniform Terminology for Reporting Occupational Therapy Services.* Rockville, MD: AOTA, 1978

5. Mosey AC: A model for occupational therapy. *Occupational Therapy in Mental Health.* New York: The Haworth Press, 1980, pp 11-29

6. Reilly M: A psychiatric occupational therapy program as a teaching model. *Am J Occup Ther* 20: 66-67, 1966

7. Clark PN: Human development through occupation: A philosophy and conceptual model for practice, part 2. *Am J Occup Ther* 33: 577-585, 1979

8. Shannon PD: Work-play theory and the occupational process. *Am J Occup Ther* 26: 169-172, 1972

9. Sharp C: *The Economics of Time.* New York: John Wiley and Sons, 1981

10. de Grazia S: *Of Time, Work, and Leisure.* New York: The Twentieth Century Fund, 1962

11. Douglass ME, Douglass DN: *Manage Your Time, Manage Your Work, Manage Yourself.* New York: AMACOM 1980

12. Cox MH, Shepard RJ: Employee fitness, absenteeism, and job satisfaction. *Med and Sci in Sports,* 11: 105, 1979

13. Durbeck DC: The National Aeronautics and Space Administration U.S. Public Health Service health evaluation and enhancement program. *Am J Card,* 30: 788-9, 1972

14. Haskell WL, Blair SN: The physical activity component of health promotion in occupational settings. *Public Health Reports,* 29: 109-118, 1980

15. Morris JN: Coronary heart disease and physical activity of work. *Lancet,* 2: 1053-57, 1953

16. Brunner D., Manelis G: Myocardial infarction among members of communal settlements in Israel. *Lancet,* 2: 1049, 1960

17. Fox SM, Naughton JP, Haskell WL: Physical activity and the prevention of coronary heart disease. *Annals of Clinical Research,* 3: 404-32, 1973

18. Froelicher VF: The effects of chronic exercise on the heart and on coronary atherosclerotic heart disease: A literature review. *Cardiovascular Clinic,* Philadelphia: F.A. Davis, 1976

19. Paffenbarger RS, Brand RJ, Sholtz RI, Jung DL: Energy expenditure, cigarette smoking, and blood pressure level as related to death from specific disease. *Am J Ep,* 108: 12-18, 1978

20. Shapiro S, Weinblatt E, Frank CW, Soger RV: Incidence of coronary heart disease in a population insured for medical care. *Am J Pub Hlth,* 59: 100-1, 1969

21. Sehnert KW, Tillotson JK: *A National Health Care Strategy: How Business Can Promote Good Health for Employees and Their Families* Washington, D.C.: National Chamber Foundation, 1978

22. Ellwood PM, McClure WJ, Rosala J: *A National Health Care Strategy: How Business Interacts With the Health Care System,* Washington, D.C.: National Chamber Foundation, 1978

23. Harmon P: Information presented at the *Tri County Industrial Recreation Council Conference*, San Jose, CA, 1983

24. Nie NH, Hull CH, Jenkins JG, Steinbrenner K, Bent DH: *Statistical Package for the Social Sciences*, 2nd edition. New York: McGraw-Hill, 1975

25. Cantor SG: Occupational therapy and occupational medicine—A merger. *Am J Occup Ther*, 33: 631-34, 1979

26. Pelletier KR: *A Parcourse for Health Promotion Programs in the Work Place, The Final Report.* San Francisco, CA: California Nexus Foundation, 1983

27. Dempster-Ogden L: *Initial Evaluation of the Cardiac Patient—Occupational Therapy.* Downey, CA: Cardiac Rehabilitation Resources, 1981

The Expanding Role of Occupational Therapy in the Treatment of Industrial Hand Injuries

Jane Bear-Lehman, MS, OTR
Eva McCormick, OTR

ABSTRACT. A recent survey of members of the American Society of Hand Therapists revealed an expanding role for the therapist in the treatment of industrial hand injuries. In the traditional role of treatment provider, occupational therapists are using their assessment tools and work capacity programming to aid in predicting return to work readiness. This is aimed at preventing reinjury of the present patient population.

In addition to this, therapists have begun to identify relationships between specific injuries and work that produced them. This gives rise to a specified goal of preventing the injury from ever occurring. To reach this goal therapists are becoming involved in industrial settings and are working with industrial safety teams.

INTRODUCTION

Upper extremity injuries are a major cause of disability, affecting persons in their wage earning years. U.S. statistics show that of the total number of injuries incurred in industrial and agricultural work, one third affect the upper extremity.[1] This high incidence has a significant economic impact on work time lost and on medical costs.

Jane Bear-Lehman, formerly a Consultant in Hand Therapy to Henry Bernstein, MD, Ltd. in Elmwood Park IL; currently an Assistant Professor in Occupational Therapy at the University of Toronto, Toronto, Ontario, Canada.

Eva McCormick, Director of Occupational Therapy at Foster G. McGaw Hospital of Loyola University, Maywood, IL.

The authors extend thanks to the American Society of Hand Therapists and its members who shared their return to work programs through our survey.

This article appears jointly in *Work-Related Programs in Occupational Therapy* (The Haworth Press, 1985) and *Occupational Therapy in Health Care,* Volume 2, Number 4 (Winter 1985/1986).

79

A report published in 1982 stated that each worker who suffered an upper extremity injury was away from the job for an average of 17 days.[2] Such work accidents involving the upper extremity cost over ten billion dollars annually.[3]

Many workers in industrial factories are at risk to injure their hands with the tools they use or on the machines they operate. Sudden impact injuries can be caused by any one of the 290,000 power presses, 455,000 drill presses, 280,000 milling machines, and 195,000 cut off saws in the U.S.[3] Statistics are now also being collected on the more silent hand injuries, the cumulative trauma disorders.[4] These injuries are produced over time and are caused by the use of poorly designed tools and work stations or improper work performance movements.[5] Incidence data on the cumulative trauma disorders is difficult to gather as the disease definition is inconsistent and often the diagnosis is not reported. The workmen's compensation and legal systems have not yet accepted that cumulative trauma may be occupationally produced.[6]

The U.S. Department of Labor and the U.S. Consumer Products Safety Commission have been documenting how accidents occur. In the last decade labor unions have become involved in safety and health issues, and mobilized support to pass the Occupational Safety and Health Act (OSHA) of 1970.[7] The Act replaced the privately controlled compensation-safety apparatus that had existed in the U.S. since 1910. The Occupational Safety and Health Act governs an administrative division within the U.S. Department of Labor devoted to reducing hazards in the work place.

There has been a slight reduction in overall work injuries which can be attributed to OSHA's unannounced factory inspection tours and to the increased use of protective equipment now required in the work place.[8] The OSHA system has been under continual political scrutiny concerning its areas of concentration and its recommendations to the work place. Its mission is vast; operating under severe budgetary and manpower shortages, it can be equated to a band-aid over a large open wound.

Despite the large number of occupational injuries, the U.S. Department of Labor confirms that effective prevention is practiced in many work places, and that nearly one-half of all work places report no recordable injuries in a year's time.[9] Commitment from both management and labor in industry is needed to identify existing occupational hazards, and to work with engineers, ergonomists, physicians, and therapists in preventing injuries in areas where they are continually produced.

It has been shown that educating industrial plant supervisors and redesigning both tools and work stations are essential in the reduction of hand injuries.[10] The medical community can be influential in injury prevention by work with local safety and industrial groups to develop educational programs and to investigate injuries.[11] Therapists' and surgeons' knowledge of bodily mechanics, postures, and tolerances can be valuable input for a safety job analysis.

The occupational therapist is trained to measure the physical, social, and psychological effects of activity on an individual. The purpose of this paper is to identify the therapist's role in prevention, and to explore how the role has expanded to interface with the industrial community. Survey results from the members of the American Society of Hand Therapists will be used to illustrate the current direction of this role.

PREVENTION

Prevention is often divided into two levels: primary prevention and secondary.[12] Primary prevention aims to prevent the injury-producing event from occurring. Prevention is becoming an integral part of medical practice and comprehensive health care. To address primary prevention the occupational therapist must either expand or shift from the role of treatment provider to that of researcher/practitioner working to prevent initial occurrences.[12,13] In such a role the occupational therapist identifies the existence of preventable conditions and works with researchers to trace retrospectively the effect back to the cause. The ability to bring about changes in accident prone environments is directly related to blocking the cause-effect relationship.

Wilma West defines second stage of prevention as ''early detection of disease, deficit, deviation, dysfunction, and disability followed by appropriate intervention to prevent progression to more serious or chronic condition''.[14] This definition suggests a screening process for early intervention which precedes rehabilitation. This level of prevention is not as new for occupational therapists as is the first level, primary prevention.

Working on prevention is not for every occupational therapist.[12,13] To take part in prevention, the therapist must be willing to learn about the worker's job and become familiar with the worker's compensation and related legal systems. The therapist must feel comfortable in this shift in focus from acute care practitioner in an medical environment to that of practitioner/researcher advocating prevention needs.[12,15]

PRE-VOCATIONAL ASSESSMENT AND PREVENTION

Historically, occupational therapists have worked as primary treatment agents facilitating rehabilitation for persons with hand injury.[12] The therapist strives to help them achieve maximum use of their hands for both avocational and vocational activities. To minimize the risk of reinjury upon return to work, therapists have begun to evaluate their patients' abilities to perform job related activities in the therapy clinic. Many therapists compare the results of their patient's physical capacity assessment to the job requirements. Therapy then aims to bridge the gap between the capacity that the patient possesses and the physical demands of the job. This type of program offers a classical second stage level of prevention.

With advanced surgical techniques and therapeutic skills, more hands are being saved and restored. Return to work is expected by the patient, by the treatment team, and by society. The treatment team, which includes the physician, therapist, and patient, assesses the readiness of the patient to return to work and the ability to perform his job safely. Many therapists have been developing prevocational assessment batteries to predict readiness for return to work.[16,17] Treatment programs to develop work skills and endurance have also appeared.[16,17] Many of these programs resemble the prevocational procedures available to occupational therapists in the 1950's but implement 1980 technology. An example of this is the Baltimore Therapeutic Equipment (BTE) Work Simulator which is a compact instrument designed to provide specific repetitive upper limb motions against measurable resistances over a specified amount of time. It quantitatively documents the work output of the user.[21]

ACTIVITIES OF THE AMERICAN SOCIETY OF HAND THERAPISTS

The American Society of Hand Therapists (ASHT) is comprised of occupational and physical therapists who have specialized in the rehabilitation of the hand. Concerned with the development of education and research in safety and the prevention of hand injuries, ASHT formed a special task force in 1981 to study the role of hand therapy in safety and prevention. The task force reported that there were few published studies on the prevention of hand injuries.[22] However, Baxter, Matheson, and Smith advocated the broadening of the therapist's role from solely acute care to include special rehabilitation programs for the achievement of safe return to work.[16,17,23] They introduced the value of the physical capacity evaluation for directing rehabilitation goals, advocated the use of work tools and work media in the therapy environment for rehearsal and simulation of work skills, and recommended on-site job evaluations. This last recommendation suggests the formation of a new treatment team, namely, therapist-patient-employer, for facilitating the transition from medical treatment to return to work. To identify the expansion of the roles in hand therapy, members of ASHT were surveyed.

ASHT SURVEY

In 1983, a questionnaire was sent to the 200 members of the ASHT to detect practice trends in the programs geared toward the return to work of hand injured workers. The survey yielded a 40% response rate. The questionnaire gathered information on methods of assessment used, problems that impeded return to work, types of injuries treated, and types of communication networks established with other specialists for achievement of safe return to work for hand injured patients.

SURVEY RESULTS

To identify types of services and where they occur, the data were divided into three subgroups based on where treatment had occurred, that is, in hospitals, physicians' offices, or hand centers. Data showed that in all three settings the majority of patients treated had crush injuries, fractures, and tendon/nerve injuries. The average reported interval for treatment was four months, with a majority of patients concluding treatment care either in less than one month or after six months. Personnel in all 3 locations treated patients with occupations indigenous to their geographical area, with a high incidence of injured workers from construction, carpentry, printing, farming, food processing, heavy metal industry and assembly operations.

Data of subgroups showed differences in the percentages of work-related injuries as compared to other trauma and types of treatment provided. Hand centers reported that an average of 75 percent of their caseloads was work-related injuries. Physicians' offices stated that 65 percent and hospital based facilities noted that 40 percent of caseload was work-related injuries. Eighty-six percent of all the respondents indicated they provided acute care services; the remaining percentage represented hand centers that did not accept patients during the acute stage of injury. The therapists who work in physicians' offices were the only ones who tended to evaluate patients preoperatively. All subgroups provided splinting as well as exercise and activity programs directed at restoring hand function.

Several facilities reported providing specific treatment for facilitating return to work. Sixty percent cited use of job simulated tasks in treatment, 40 percent offered work hardening or conditioning tasks, and 30 percent, provided physical capacity evaluations. Job simulation and work hardening programs occurred in physicians' offices and hand centers. The overall incidence of use of physical capacity evaluations was low and equally distributed among the three subgroups. The complexity of physical capacity evaluations used, however, varied. Some incorporated the work of Matheson or Smith and some were of independent design.[17,23] Others included on-site visits to the job combined with the BTE work simulator or used only the work simulator.[21] In all kinds of facilities, the respondents indicated that the hand therapists who were occupational therapists administered the return to work evaluations and directed the work hardening treatment.

Several respondents observed relationships between the upper extremity injury and the machine, tool, or industrial task that produced them. Therapists noted the cause and effect relationship between a given industry and specific types of injuries. In some instances the therapists were able to establish liaison with industry in order to work together in prevention programs. Information about injury prevention has been shared with industrial management personnel and workers in lectures which focused on proper body mechanics and in the use of safety devices. Therapists also reported the use of this industrial contact to discuss concerns for returning an injured worker to the job.

DISCUSSION

Since 1981 the interest in and the inclusion of return to work programming in the rehabilitation phase of hand treatment has mushroomed. This is exemplified by the content of recent ASHT conferences and by the appearance of several private practices for assessing return to work readiness. Also programs for work evaluation and work hardening are proliferating across the country.

The new frontier of first level prevention continues to be carved with therapists and surgeons teaming up with industrial engineers, ergonomic specialists, and industrial safety managers. Efforts to reduce work related hand injuries continue to grow in inter-disciplinary conferences such as those by the Chicago Safety Council.[11] Also, Dr. Sidney Blair, a hand surgeon, working within the Chicago Area Safety Council had been instrumental in studying the incidence of industrial accidents in the power press industry.[11] The joint interest between Medicine and the power press industry initiated several local workshops.

The role of the hand therapist in safety and prevention includes the identification of high risk tasks and equipment. Douglas, Slack and several ASHT survey respondents have linked specific injuries to particular industries or machines as shown in Figure 1.[24,25] Tenosynovitis and carpal tunnel syndrome have been associated with the use of crimpers in micro-assembly and electronics. Some therapists have begun to work directly with industries to diminish the incidence of hand injuries; they have introduced favorable work postures and have established preventive strengthening exercise programs.

Professionals involved in the goal of returning injured workers to jobs have included such disciplines as rehabilitation nurses, hand therapists, hand surgeons, industrial commissioners, worker's compensation lawyers, and other representatives from industry. Seminars continue to appear at power press industry meetings to emphasize the impact of press injuries in terms of the enormity of problems in surgical repair from the resultant crush injuries and the long term rehabilitation required. Other seminars involving ergonomists and safety engineers have also been held to discuss repetitive motion disease, that is, injury that can result to various tissues in the body as a result of cumulative mechanical trauma over time.[26]

CONCLUSION

A major emphasis in treatment continues to be primary therapeutic care for the injured hand. Interest, not only in doing but in perfecting return to work assessment, however, has grown among therapists in magnitude and intensity.[12] In the study of ASHT members

INDUSTRIAL TASK/OCCUPATION	TYPE OF INJURY
printing rollers press work: (punch, loom, jewelry) tank hatch: (military) conveyor belts farm machinery	crush injury
corn picker	traumatic amputation
processing; (meat, poultry) repetitive crimping tools repetitive assembly jack hammers	carpal tunnel syndrome
glass work butcher wood working: saws	tendon/nerve damage
dentist/nurse	cellulitis
writers, secretaries hospital aids dieticians	dequervain's

Figure 1: The relationship between industrial tasks and occupations and types of hand injuries.

reported, it was the hand therapist/occupational therapist who was identified most often as the return to work evaluator and treatment coordinator. Services aimed at safely determining the timing and the needs for return to work of patients with hand injuries have also expanded. This expansion focuses attention on secondary level prevention, that is, minimizing the risk of additional injury. This focus on safe and appropriate return to work of injured persons serves to establish working communications between personnel at both medical treatment facilities and industrial sites.

Therapists, nonetheless, continue to search for the best tool or collection of tools to assess physical capacity. The procedures outlined by Baxter and Smith are frequently adopted.[16,23] Some facilities have also begun to use more tool related procedures such as Matheson's W.E.S.T. or the BTE Work Simulator.[17,21] Choices of equipment and test battery as a whole vary with the size and budget of the facility as well as with the needs of the patient population. Many centers choose a collection of instruments to provide the broadest base possible for observational analysis. Unfortunately, many of the tools available to date are not standardized, and they also fall short in their capacity to predict performance reliably.

In many instances the pursuit by therapists of secondary prevention has been a logical progression in thinking. As soon as a communication link has been established between a treatment facility and a particular industry, dialogue on primary prevention can occur, with the effect of working together to prevent specific injuries from ever occurring. This evolution is often a delicate negotiation, but, if achieved, industrial and medical personnel can jointly address the issue of prevention; it also can bear significant results toward reduction of injuries. Organizational networks and symposia tend to be the focal points linking the medically concerned surgeon and therapist with the industrial community.

The occupational therapist's unique blend of expertise in occupational performance, body mechanics, along with the ability to teach both joint protection and work simplification principles is of great value to an industrial prevention program. In addition to this, the occupational therapist can use knowledge of anatomy, physiology, as well as understanding of the processes of disease and injury to identify the right activities and exercise procedures to increase the workers' strength and endurance, and to minimize the effect of their required postures and work patterns. The need for occupational therapists to expand their services into the area of prevention is not a new concept.[14] The growing demand however for such activity in assisting injured workers to return to full employment is a prime opportunity. That path is beginning to be firmly established by a few.

REFERENCES

1. Kelsey JL, Pastides H, Kreiger N: *Upper Extremity Disorders*, St. Louis: The CV Mosby Company, 1980
2. U.S. Department of Labor: Work-related hand injuries and upper extremity amputations. Bureau of Labor Statistics. Bulletin 2160, Washington, DC, 1982
3. *Accident facts*, Chicago, Illinois: National Safety Council, 1980
4. Armstrong TJ, Foulke JA, Joseph BS and Goldstein SA: Investigation of cumulative

trauma disorders in a poultry processing plant. *American Ind. Hyg. Assoc. J.* 43:103-116, 1982

5. Meagher, SW: Human factors engineering: A primer for the surgeon's participation in industrial injury prevention. *Contemporary Orthopaedics,* 8:73-80, 1984

6. Hadler, NM *Medical Management of the Regional Musculoskeletal Diseases,* Toronto: Grune and Stratton, Inc., 1984

7. Berman D. *Death on the Job,* New York: Monthly Review Press, 1978

8. OSHA: Occupational Health and Safety Act

9. Leads from the MMWR, *JAMA,* 251:2503-2504, 1984

10. Kuorinka I: Repetitive Tasks, Presented at Task Injury Workshop, New York, 1984

11. Blair SJ and Allard KM: Prevention of trauma: a cooperative effort. *J of Hand Surg,* 8:649-53, 1983

12. Stein F: Occupational therapy services in prevention of illness. *Am J Occ Ther,* 33:225-6, 1977

13. Cantor SG: Occupational therapy and occupational medicine—a merger, *Am J Occ Ther,* 33:631-4, 1979

14. West WA: The growing importance of prevention. *Am J Occ Ther,* 23:226-231, 1969

15. Blair SJ, Bear-Lehman J, McCormick EH: Industrial hand injuries; prevention and rehabilitation. In *Rehabilitation of the Hand,* 2nd Edition, Hunter, Schneider, Editors. St. Louis: The CV Mosby Company, 1984

16. Baxter PL and Fried SL: The work tolerance program of the Hand Rehabilitation Centre in Philadelphia. In *Rehabilitation of the Hand,* 2nd Edition, Hunter, Schneider, Editors. St. Louis: CV Mosby Company, 1984

17. Matheson LN: *Work capacity evaluation,* Trabuco Canyon, California: Rehabilitation Institute of Southern California, 1982

18. Cromwell F: A procedure for prevocational evaluation, *Am J Occ Ther,* 13(1) 1-4, 1959

19. Wegg LS: The essentials of work evaluation, *Am J Occ Ther,* 14(2) 65-69, 1960

20. Reuss EE, Rauk DE, Sundquist AE: Development of a physical capabilities evaluation, *Am J Occ Ther,* 12(1) 1-8, 1958

21. Curtis RM, Clark GL, Snyder A: The work simulator. In *Rehabilitation of the Hand,* 2nd Edition, Hunter, Schneider, Editors. St. Louis: CV Mosby Company, 1984

22. McCormick EH: Safety and Prevention Committee Report. *Newsletter of the American Society of Hand Therapists,* 3:9, 1983

23. Smith SL: Physical capacity evaluation. In *Willard and Spackman's Occupational Therapy,* Sixth Edition, Hopkins and Smith, Editors. Philadelphia: The JD Lippincott Company, 1978

24. Douglas JR: Grant Hospital of Chicago Work Capacity Program. *Newsletter of the American Society of Hand Therapists,* 3:9, 1983

25. Slack DA: Occupational therapy in industrial rheumatology, presented at AOTA Annual Conference, Philadelphia, 1982

26. Armstrong TJ: Evaluation and design of jobs for control of cumulative trauma disorders. Presented at Cumulative Trauma Disorders of the Upper Extremity Symposium, Ann Arbor, Michigan, 1984

PRACTICE WATCH:

Things for Leaders and Managers to Think About

Occupational Therapy Leadership Potential Can Be Developed Through Marketing Techniques

Grace E. Gilkeson, EdD, OTR, FAOTA

Accountability and competition are becoming key words with which to characterize occupational therapy practice today, yet these words have been relatively rare in the professional vocabulary of therapists. Now occupational therapists are being faced with the demands these words imply and are finding them linked with survival as everyday realities. Occupational therapists who operate in highly competitive climates are concerned about duplication and overlap with other services as well as being able to justify occupational therapy.

Those persons responsible for funding health care today are sophisticated judges of management and efficiency. They are now holding all health care providers to high standards of management and function. Federal and state governments are making demands in the form of additional regulatory requirements. Increasingly enlightened, educated consumers are adding their own justified, rightful demands when they seek occupational therapy services. Therapists in private practice find new tax and business responsibilities. New and changing roles and locations of practices are commonplace as occupational therapists respond to changing health care needs.

How can occupational therapists cope with such forces and succeed in a climate of competition? It is suggested that occupational therapists can better compete if they take more responsibility for marketing their own services, for assuming more risks in program development, for learning more non-treatment skills as they think, act, and manage themselves to meet these new demands. This includes

Grace E. Gilkeson is Dean, School of Occupational Therapy, Texas Women's University, Denton, TX.

This article appears jointly in *Work-Related Programs in Occupational Therapy* (The Haworth Press, 1985) and Occupational Therapy in Heatlh Care, Volume 2, Number 4 (Winter 1985/1986).

developing a marketing attitude by systematically and realistically investigating the needs of all with whom daily transactions are conducted.

The social, economic, and political pressures today require reassessment of the occupational therapist role and planning of strategies for action to ensure continued growth of the occupational therapy profession. Occupational therapists must 'think marketing' daily, matching their information to the interests and needs of those whom they hope to serve and satisfy. Carefully outlining services offered on the other persons' terms is only part of the job. Occupational therapists must first believe in, understand, and be able to clearly describe their product—occupational therapy—before they can make judgments about new and advantageous applications. Exactly what service/product is being offered? The position held by occupational therapy in the highly competitive and increasingly fragmented marketplace must be determined, decisions made about market segments, then careful plans made to proceed.

Marketing skills are closely aligned with those of leadership. Both are essential to the future of occupational therapy, to be sure, and the techniques of each can be learned and practiced by those who choose to control their own futures. Public relations is more than advertising, and marketing is more than selling. Both are important, and both require analytic thought, constant planning, feedback and evaluation of the needs to be met as well as the services designed to meet them.

Marketing may also be considered as an example of successful application of the systems approach. Stated simply, the marketing process applied to a current occupational therapy problem would involve a structured series of procedures. For example, you need first to state your specific problem, determine all the constituencies/publics involved, identify present and potential exchanges, evaluate the environments, and estimate the status of the market. Having established this background, you will next focus on determination of the constituents which represent feasible markets and outline your market segments and opportunities. Finally, select your strategy, decide which segments warrant priority attention and how much, and evaluate each one while estimating the competition. After implementing your strategy, re-evaluation and readjustment of your approach is suggested, much as one would perceive the feedback loops in a systems approach. To become leaders within the health care delivery system today, occupational therapists must develop a systematic evaluative marketing attitude such as described. Charles Farrell gives us food for thought by stating that, "a tiger who does not prowl is a potential rug."

From still another perspective usable by occupational therapists in administrative positions, marketing is a major policy-making function which belongs in all levels of management. It basically leads to decisions about what services to offer, whom to serve and how, and issues of pricing, referral and how services are accessed. Marketing is a function commonly found in for-profit businesses but heretofore not in most traditional health care provider organizations. The language and techniques germane to marketing can be learned and applied to practice by occupational therapists in the context of today's changing health care environments. They would thus be enabled to promote services, increase referrals, improve image and visibility, and compete successfully. Understanding the marketing process gives occupational therapists the tools necessary to accomplish ever-changing goals.

Growing numbers of occupational therapists are employed as health care team members both in institutional and community practice. With excellent generalist backgrounds and flexible approaches, occupational therapists are eminently well-qualified to serve as leaders of these interdisciplinary teams. Occupational therapists are trained to globally assess the total person, to utilize interpersonal skills.

Like most health care providers occupational therapists until now have usually delivered services which they themselves professionally deemed necessary. This might be known as a non-marketing approach to planning and development and is exactly opposite to a true marketing approach. MacStravic (1977) suggested that organizations or providers should identify what the public perceives as its needs, determine which of those needs the organization is best equipped and able to meet effectively and efficiently, and develop high quality services and programs based on such estimations. Not only can quality be increased, but the occupational therapist using a marketing approach will also find quantity of services positively affected. Since problems of accountability must be addressed daily, marketing offers a viable assist in this dilemma. Both marketing and non-marketing approaches are based on meeting needs, but each has a different definition and method of measuring needs. Occupational therapy and all of health care today demand a marketing approach! How else can the direction of future practice be guided?

Finally, occupational therapists may well find their services growing in both use and acceptance if they are willing to apply a few ideas suggested here:

1. Recognition and use of the similarities among the concepts of marketing, public relations and leadership in planning and delivering services.
2. Application of marketing principles and techniques to their occupational therapy practice.
3. Analysis of present and potential populations able to benefit from their unique occupational therapy services.
4. Development of marketing plans for specific populations in need of these services.
5. Implementation of marketing plans with evaluation and feedback.

As headlined in a recent issue of *U.S. News and World Report,* "Marketing is the Name of the Game for the 80s." In marketing, occupational therapists can find one strategy that will support the continued growth of their services in the decade ahead. Now is the time to become marketing specialists.

REFERENCE

MacStravic, Robin E. (1977). *Marketing health care.* Germantown: Aspen.

Time Management
in Clinical Practice

Peter M. Talty, MS, OTR

ABSTRACT. Organizing one's time to accomplish the tasks that bombard an occupational therapist each day is imperative to personal and professional survival. Clinicians have more and greater responsibility than ever before, but are not able to quantitatively increase the number of clock hours to handle the increased workload. The answer lies in managing one's allocated time more effectively.

Clincians can fall into the same "time traps" as everyone else. They can waste time by not concentrating on one task at a time, or through procrastination. It is not unusual for a clinician to attempt to see as many patients as possible without a clear system of priority setting.

This article outlines ways of applying time management principles to the unique demands of clinical practice. Specific methods of increasing a clinician's time management skills are presented through the Clinical Time Log, the System of Clinical Prioritization, applications of Pareto's Rule, and specific suggestions for better time management in clinical practice.

INTRODUCTION

According to the Health Care Financing Administration, $355 billion was spent for health care in the United States in 1983 amounting 10.8% of the gross national product. These figures represent a

Peter Talty received both his bachelors and masters degrees from the State University of New York at Buffalo, his bachelors in Occupational Therapy and masters in Health Sciences Education. He has utilized his education and training in various supervisory and managerial positions with several New York State health care facilities. At present he is Vice President of Patient Care Services, Bry-Lin Hospital in Buffalo, New York.

In addition to full-time clinical and administrative responsibilities at Bry-Lin, he holds academic appointments on the faculties of Erie Community College and the State University of New York at Buffalo. His areas of special interest include managing stress at home and on the job, problem solving and decision making in management, effective communication, and time management.

This article appears jointly in *Work-Related Programs in Occupational Therapy* (The Haworth Press, 1985) and *Occupational Therapy in Health Care*, Volume 2, Number 4 (Winter 1985/1986).

95

10.3% increase over 1982 expenditures.[1] Efforts to control the escalating costs of delivering health care have included Diagnostic Related Groupings (DRG's), Preferred Provider Organizations (PPO's), and other fiscal mandates to enhance more cost-effective operations. The productivity of the clinical practitioners who provide health services is a controllable factor in the total cost of health care. Increasing the individual productivity of clinical staff through more effective time management practices can contribute to cost containment without a decrease in the quality of services provided.

This article will review selected time management principles and discuss the application of these principles to the delivery of clinical service. The time management principles and techniques to be discussed are: the Clinical Time Log, Clinical Prioritization, Pareto's Rule, Prime Time, and High Yield Performance. Although time management principles are applicable to all disciplines engaged in delivering a clinical service, the emphasis in this article will be on the field of occupational therapy.

CLINICAL TIME LOG

The Clinical Time Log is a tool which will assist clinicians in determining: (1) How time is currently utilized? (2) How does actual time distribution compare with optimal time distribution? (3) How does the actual time distribution compare with the emphasis in the job description? (4) What impact does the actual time distribution have on clinical productivity?

The Log provides space for recording of tasks performed in half-hour blocks of time for five working days. All "working" time is sub-divided into six categories: (See Figure 1):

1. *Direct Service Time* (D) Time spent providing direct clinical service to patients or their families in a face-to-face relationship. Activities included in this category are observing, testing, interviewing, assessing, evaluating, treating, training, counseling, educating, or motivating patients or their families.
2. *Indirect Service Time* (I) Time spent in formulating treatment plans, analyzing and interpreting results of evaluations, documenting results of evaluations and treatments, reviewing records, conferring with colleagues, reviewing literature, or attending case conferences.

3. *Supervisory Time* (S) Time spent in supervising staff, students, or volunteers. Specifically, time spent recruiting, interviewing, selecting, orienting, training, reprimanding, evaluating, motivating, or terminating staff, students, or volunteers.
4. *Administrative Time* (A) Time spent in writing or reading policies, procedures, memos, reports, forms, or attending non-clinical meetings.
5. *Self-Development Time* (SD) Time spent in increasing one's knowledge or skills by reading professional literature or by attending inservices, workshops, or conferences.
6. *Service to One's Profession Time* (SP) Time spent in promoting or developing one's profession by attending meetings, running for and holding an office, serving on committees, doing research, publishing, and the conducting of workshops and seminars.

Excluded from the Log is "non-working" time including lunch, coffee breaks, and other forms of recovery periods. The Log's focus is on service and service-related time.

During a typical two-week period, each clinician records his time on the Log utilizing the key provided. Since the activities engaged in during a given half-hour block may be varied, the number of minutes engaged in the activity is recorded in parentheses next to the letter. Entries are recorded as soon as possible to enhance the accuracy of the finished Log.

At the end of each day the totals are recorded on the Clinical Time Log Summary (see Figure 2). The working time of each day is then totaled in minutes for each time category.

UTILIZATION OF CLINICAL TIME LOG DATA

The completed Log serves as a feedback mechanism for clinicians, supervisors, and administrators. There should be a correlation between the job description and actual distribution of time utilization. Distortions occur, for example, when a clinician's direct Service Time has been reduced to less than 30% of the total working time available. When actual time and activities engaged in are no longer reflected in a job description, adjustments are needed. Adjustments can be made in the job description or the staff members responsibilities and assignments.

FIGURE 1.

CLINICAL TIME LOG

Dates: From: ____ To: ____	TIME CATEGORIES: KEY D = Direct Service Time I = Indirect Service Time S = Supervisory Time A = Administrative Time SD = Self-Development Time SP = Service to one's Profession Time				
DAY TIME	MONDAY	TUESDAY	WEDNESDAY	THURSDAY	FRIDAY

May be reproduced

FIGURE 2.
CLINICAL TIME LOG SUMMARY

Clinician:____________________ Dates:__________ To____________

DAY / TIME CATEGORY	MON	TUES	WED	THUR	FRI	TOTALS BY CATEGORY
(D) DIRECT SERVICE TIME						
(I) INDIRECT SERVICE TIME						
(S) SUPERVISORY TIME						
(A) ADMINISTRATI. TIME						
(SD) SELF-DEVELOPMENT TIME						
(SP) SERVICE TO ONE'S PROFESSION T.						
TOTALS BY DAY						

May be reproduced

The demands of clinical practice can often lead to frustration for a practitioner who is providing less service than preferred. Through completion of the Clinical Time Log, all concerned have data that accurately reflects present operations. Patterns and trends can be identified and corrective measures taken if warranted. The results of the completed Clinical Time Log Summary serve as a control device for supervisors, and the basis for supervisory counseling sessions. The amount of time to be spent in each category will vary depending upon the setting, caseload, job title, and responsibilities outlined in the job description.

SETTING PRIORITIES

Once the Clinical Time Log is completed and analyzed, the next step is to set priorities on tasks and responsibilities. Through a process of negotiation between supervisors and clinicians, and using the Log Summary as the data base, the process of prioritization begins.

A systematic method of setting clinical priorities is based on Alan Lakein's ABC Priority System. According to Lakein, not all of the tasks on a list of things to do have the same value. An "A" is an item on the list that is urgent and has high value. A "B" is one with medium or high value, but is not as urgent as the "A". Low value items are considered to be "C's". By value, Lakein is referring to the person's estimate of the relative value of each item to that person.

Establishing priorities can result in conflicts between the expectations of the position and those of the clinician. Indirect Service versus Direct Service is a frequent conflict area. Writing progress notes or treating patients is an example of this conflict in practice. Resolving such conflicts can be difficult.

An example of applying the ABC's to clinical practice from occupational therapy can be seen in Figure 3. The A's, B's, and C's are based on criteria established for an acute care hospital. Time may not permit all patients to receive the same extent of occupational therapy services. Therefore, by establishing criteria, a systematic method of determining clinical priorities results.

It is suggested that each facility establish a System of Clinical Prioritization specific to their operation. The System should be known by all staff, and revised as needed.

PARETO'S RULE IN CLINICAL PRACTICE

Vilfredo Pareto, the 19th century economist and sociologist, offers a principle that can further the process of priority setting. According to Pareto, "the significant items in a given group normally

FIGURE 3.

SYSTEM OF CLINICAL PRIORITIZATION FOR AN ACUTE
CARE HOSPITAL'S OCCUPATIONAL THERAPY SERVICE

PRIOR.	CRITERIA (Examples only)	CLINICAL EXAMPLES
A's	Patients experiencing pain that could be alleviated through proper joint alignment with a splint.	Rheumatoid Arthritis during inflammatory stage.
	Patients who can be independent in a brief period.	High functioning patient with Hemiplegia
	Patients at high risk for contractures.	Burns
	Patients who can have an abbreviated length of inpatient stay.	ADL training of mild CVA.
B's	Patients prone to contracture but not at immediate risk.	Stabilized patient with CVA.
	Patients requiring substantial treatment or training to produce independence.	Parkinson's Disease
	Patients with deficits in strength due to progressive condition.	Multiple Sclerosis
C's	Patients whose disabilities are of such severity or multiplicity that the functional prognosis is extremely poor.	Patients who are acutely medically ill.
	Patients who lack the cognitive ability to comprehend even the lowest level of information.	Advanced Alzheimer's Disease
	Patients whose condition is chronic and have shown no motivation.	Paraplegia of long duration.

constitute a relatively small portion of the total items in the group.'' Stated another way, all tasks to be done on a given ''To Do List'' do not have the same (e.g., ''A'') value. There are a few tasks that, if completed, will yield a high return on the investment of one's time. Pareto's Rule has some interesting applications to clinical practice when combined with the System of Clinical Prioritization.

Not all patients on a clinician's caseload are going to respond equally to the rehabilitation process. Some are highly motivated, have accepted their disability, are intact cognitively, and work in tandem with the clinician to achieve treatment goals. Others will respond and progress if given the time and caring of a supportive environment. The final grouping are those patients that, in spite of time and the best of services, do not achieve treatment goals.

Caseloads can be prioritized utilizing Pareto's Rule and the System of Clinical Prioritization. Clinical judgement plays a major role in this type of decision making and clinicians with more experience will need to assist the less experienced clinicians. The questions that can guide the clinician in determining clinical priorities include but are not limited to:

1. Which patients in the caseload have the greatest potential for recovery and independence?
2. Do the above patients have the ''tools'' for rehabilitation (motivation, cognition, etc.)?
3. Which patients have, or have not, demonstrated the drive for independence?

DANGERS OF CLINICAL PRIORITIZATION

Any system of categorization runs the risk of reducing people to a list of characteristics without full appreciation for the human potential factor. Categorization can also lead to oversimplification of complex processes. Therefore, patients should not be categorized as ''C's'' in terms of potential to benefit from rehabilitation and then never be expected to rise above staffs' expectations. This would not be the proper use of the Clinical Prioritization System. The Clinical Prioritization System is meant to be a flexible guide to aid clinicians in identifying patients who will benefit the greatest from the investment of a clinician's time, energy, knowledge, and skill.

The Pareto Rule can also apply to the general scope of clinical responsibilities. For a department head, the provision of clinical service is usually not the primary purpose of the position. However, a staff therapist has the delivering of clinical service as the main focus of activity. Tasks need to be reviewed for each position and clear directives issued to the persons occupying each position on the priorities. Concentrating clinical staff's time on Direct Service is the usual mode of operation. However, the multiple other tasks need to be categorized into one of the six time categories, and the commensurate weighting assigned for each staff member.

PRIME TIME AND PROCRASTINATION

Prime time is the time of day when a person is at their best. During prime time, a person has more patience and tolerance, has the ability to problem solve more effectively, and has the mental and physical energy to sustain action on a given task. The ideal arrangement is to match one's prime time to the most difficult task presenting itself. This may not always be possible, but the benefits are worth the time and effort in planning for this coupling as much as possible.

Clinically, the demands on a clinician's time cannot always be organized to match prime time with prime activities. However, because prime activities are usually difficult, complex, and sometimes emotionally draining, it is often the prime activities that have a high tendency for procrastination. The areas that each person procrastinates about are usually consistent over time. Each clinician should examine his work style and task preference. Of the activities that get put off, is there a consistency in the pattern? Of the activities or tasks that are put off, are any of them A's? These are patients that are "A" priority, but they may not receive the attention they need perhaps due to procrastination on the clinician's part. One way to overcome clincial procrastination is to schedule the tasks, patients, or activities that are particularly difficult and prone to procrastination into the clinician's prime time as much as possible.

SUGGESTIONS TO MAXIMIZE CLINICAL TIME

To maximize the utilization of one's time, the clinician would do well to incorporate the following rules into his approach to his clinical practice:

1. Organize clinical space for maximum utilization of efficiency. Having equipment in working order, the necessary supplies available, and an organized system of patient transportation and scheduling increases operational efficiency.
2. Remove clutter from desk, files, and clinic.
3. Use a daily "To Do List" prioritized according to Pareto's Rule. Generate a list of tasks without concern for prioritization.
4. Prioritize a caseload and responsibilities by using Pareto's Rule.
5. Conduct a Clinical Time Log at least annually.
6. Conquer procrastination by working on difficult tasks during prime time as much as possible.
7. Aim for consistency between one's role or job description, and one's actual consumption of time by categories.
8. Categorize all clinical tasks into the Clinical Prioritization System.
9. Remember that the breaking of old habits and the adopting of new ones requires a great deal of energy and concentration.

SUMMARY

Effective time management is a skill and requires practice to acquire. Clinicians who have not acquired effective time management skills need to examine their use of time from a strengths and weaknesses perspective. Concentrating one's energy in time management builds skills that result in an increase in a clinician's discretionary time. Discretionary time is the time individuals control and utilize according to their preferences. By utilizing one's uncontrollable time more effectively, clinicians can work on the tasks they feel have the most value.

REFERENCES

Gibson, Robert M. et al. *Health Care Financing Review,* Vol 6, #2, Winter 1984
Lakein, Alan. *How To Get Control of Your Time and Your Life.* (New York: Signet, 1973)
Mackenzie, R. Alec. *The Time Trap.* (New York: AMACOM, 1972)
Purvis, George P. III. "How Time Management Got Me Under Control." *Hospital Financial Management.* January, 1979. p.42

Program Evaluation Research:
An Administrative Tool

Chestina Brollier, PhD, OTR, FAOTA

ABSTRACT. Program evaluation research should be viewed as an essential administrative tool. It can provide data needed by occupational therapy managers for assessing the effectiveness and efficiency of services and operations. This article will provide an overview of the purposes, types, basic steps, potential problems, and benefits of program evaluation.

The increasing demand for accountability and cost effectiveness in occupational therapy makes program evaluation research mandatory. Baum[1] emphasized the need for program evaluation and quality assurance studies, but a review of *The American Journal of Occupational Therapy* and *The Occupational Therapy Journal of Research* suggested that few of these studies are being published. The American Occupational Therapy Association has provided quality assurance workshops and The Efficacy Data Project has published some Data Briefs.[1,2] Nevertheless, because so few other reports exist of program evaluation research, an assumption can be made that occupational therapy managers may be unfamiliar with the process and diverse methods applicable in evaluation research.

Despite some similarities, program evaluation and quality assurance studies are distinct entities. Program evaluation uses scientific research methodologies to focus primarily on patient outcome variables as they relate to type of service, level of staff effort, cost of modality, cost of unit of service or comparative cost-effectiveness, for example.[3] In contrast, quality assurance relies heavily on peer review methods for the assessment and regulation of service

Chestina Brollier, Assistant Professor, Occupational Therapy Department, Virginia Commonwealth University, Richmond, VA.

This article appears jointly in *Work-Related Programs In Occupational Therapy* (The Haworth Press, 1985) and *Occupational Therapy in Health Care*, Volume 2, Number 4 (Winter 1985/1986).

delivery in order to satisfy accepted standards of practice developed by professional organizations and service providers.[3] Green and Attkisson[3] have provided one of the most complete definitions of program evaluation research. They believe that evaluation involves reporting the systematic collection and analysis of data in an appropriate and timely manner to assist stakeholders in judging a program's worth relative to the following criteria: (1) appropriateness of design, (2) level of effort, (3) size and nature of effects, (4) match of effects with needs, (5) cost-effectiveness, (6) strength of causal connections, and (7) use of findings for further program development, administration, planning, accountability, and advocacy.

Throughout the literature, the terms program evaluation research, evaluation research, program evaluation, and evaluation have been used interchangeably. The following will be an introduction to the purposes, types, basic steps, potential problems, and benefits of program evaluation research. Even though an occupational therapy administrator may need to hire a consultant to design and implement evaluation projects, program evaluation should be viewed as an essential administrative task. The manager should know what research questions need to be addressed by the evaluation and how to use evaluation findings to determine staff needs, costs, program objectives, and appropriateness of services.[4]

THE RELATION OF EVALUATION TO PROGRAMMING

Ideally, evaluation is built into treatment programming. Program evaluation is a tool that can enable managers to make reliable decisions about present and future departmental operations and services.[4] Feedback about successes and failures of operations and programs can enable managers and staff to monitor their work, assess their effectiveness, and make appropriate changes. By integrating evaluation into general departmental operations, the failure of one treatment method will not preclude successful operation of the department. It will instead allow for planned changes in occupational therapy services or operations. Thus, more successful outcomes in the future may follow. Essential to the use of program evaluation data is early and continual involvement of the staff and administrative personnel in planning and implementing the study. By providing input at all stages of the research process, the occupational therapy manager and staff can increase the study's relevance to their needs.

PURPOSES OF EVALUATION

Program evaluation is the application of research designs and methods to answering such questions as how successful a program or one of its parts is in fulfilling program objectives, what effects the program is having, how results are achieved, or whether the program is performing as expected. Six major purposes of program evaluation include the following: (1) to discover whether and how well program and treatment objectives are being met, (2) to determine the reasons for specific program successes and failures, (3) to uncover the principles that explain the success of a program, (4) to direct the course of experiments with treatment methods, (5) to lay the basis for further research, and (6) to redefine the means to be used for attaining objectives.[5,6,7] Program evaluation research can provide information for the following types of managerial decisions:

1. whether to accept or reject a particular treatment method used with specific patients
2. whether to continue a particular service
3. whether to institute a particular service in another part of a facility or with another patient group
4. whether to reallocate staff and/or resources to other parts of the program.

TYPES OF EVALUATION

Evaluation research can be divided into two major types although some authors include a third type for measuring program efficiency.[6,7,8,9] The two major types, which are not mutually exclusive, are called process/formative, on the one hand, and, on the other hand, either product, outcome, or summative. The questions raised and the organizational demands and resources often dictate whether one or both types are used. A process evaluation focuses on a program's operation or what is happening in the program while a product evaluation often uses experimental or quasi-experimental research designs to evaluate programming outcomes. Product evaluations can determine what the consequences of a treatment program are and if they have met desired objectives, but process evaluations are necessary to determine the details about how the results were achieved. Program evaluation, regardless of the type, should follow the rigors of scientific investigation.

Process evaluations seem to have been neglected in occupational therapy and many health care fields. There are four types of process evaluations that appear important for assessing occupational therapy treatment programs.[7,10,11] First, a *discrepancy model* compares what is written or orally described about a program's plans and objectives versus what is actually happening. This type of evaluation often uses qualitative research methods to examine the relationships between services and patients' needs or between treatment goals and services given. A *structural model* of process evaluation can be used to assess an occupational therapy department's facilities, resources, and staffing patterns. The use of client-to-staff ratios to help evaluate potential program effectiveness is included here. A *systems model* can examine the way resources are allocated. For example, time and motion studies can use this framework. Monitoring the number of patients served is another systems-oriented process evaluation strategy. The fourth type of process evaluation, *the transactional model,* focuses on unanticipated consequences of a program or treatment. Qualitative, exploratory research methods are often used to examine the positive and negative consequences that may arise from reorganization, the addition of new staff, or other sources of change and disruption in treatment programming.

In contrast to process evaluations, product, outcome and summative evaluations have become popular in many health care fields.[12] Product evaluation research typically employs quasi-experimental research designs or experimental designs and attempts to achieve a high degree of internal validity.[6,7] The effectiveness or goal attainment of certain treatment programs are assessed. Product evaluations focus on the consequences of treatment.

Frequently, evaluators are asked to move beyond assessing program effectiveness to also investigating program efficiency, the costs involved in achieving program objectives.[6,7,13,14,15] Many methods have been developed for this purpose. One of the most popular is cost-benefit analysis. The relative costs of alternative means of achieving a program's objectives are assessed. The least expensive or theoretically "best" treatment program may not be favored in a cost-benefit analysis. For example, an optimal program in terms of available resources of money, personnel, time, facilities, and/or equipment may be sought. Decision-criteria must be set. As an illustration, these might include achieving a given objective with resources available.

When evaluation research is viewed as a management responsibility and built into a treatment program, multiple types of evaluation will need to be used at various times. Sometimes outcome and efficiency measures may need to be stressed to justify services and funding, but process assessments also deserve attention because of their ability to help explain why certain outcomes are effective.

STEPS IN PROGRAM EVALUATION

The following is a brief summary of the steps typically followed in program evaluation. This outline concentrates on product or outcome studies in order to simplify the issues although process and efficiency studies contain many of the same steps.

First, a hierarchy of objectives for the program needs to be written in clear, specific, and measurable terms.[6] Particularly if the evaluator is an outside consultant, the consultant will need to closely collaborate with the occupational therapy manager and staff who have knowledge of the department's structure and functioning. The hierarchy of objectives should begin with overall objectives and be refined into supporting sub-objectives or program activities. This process may continue for several levels. Informal objectives should also be recognized. According to Suchman,[9] program evaluation can be seen as demonstrating whether the objectives at each level are being successfully achieved through the treatment and management methods used.

The second step includes the selection of the program or service to be evaluated and the development of outcome measures, which are the dependent variables. The selection of these measures depends on the intent of the treatment program being assessed. Outcome measures may reflect productivity, services offered, behavior, knowledge, values, attitudes, etc.[6] Usually outcome measures focus on changes in the people receiving services, but the measures do not have to be limited to this group. In any case, the outcome measures should describe the real changes the occupational therapy services wish to produce. Often multiple outcome measures are necessary when assessing the effects of a treatment program. Reliability and validity of the outcome measures should be considered crucial in the evaluation process.

Step three includes the identification of independent and intervening variables in order to determine why the outcomes have occurred. The independent variables usually consist of the services' purpose, theoretical framework, methods used, staffing, location of service, length of service, as well as characteristics of those being served.[6,12] The major intervening variables are program operation variables that describe the way the program functions and include patients' frequency of attendance, participation in other treatment programs, level of cooperation, family support, and the like. The particular intervening variables that should be tested in any evaluation depend upon what is being evaluated, what theoretical framework is being tested, and what is known about the field of practice from previous research and clinical experience. The occupational therapy administrator will need to collaborate with an evaluation consultant in selecting appropriate independent and intervening variables to measure because the manager has intimate knowledge of the program.

Next, a research design and data collection method must be developed and used. Because of such factors as lack of appropriate control groups or inability to manipulate the independent variables, quasi-experimental designs are often used in evaluation research. Even when true experimental designs are not used, threats to internal validity should be reduced as much as possible. The use of specific research designs and data gathering methods depends on the purpose of the evaluation and the nature of the program being assessed.

After the data have been collected and analyzed, the manager, research consultant, and staff should discuss the results and their implications. The manager can then work with the staff to develop recommendations for appropriate changes and translate recommendations into policy and procedures.[4]

PROBLEMS IN EVALUATION RESEARCH

Because program evaluation is applied research, a number of methodological problems may be encountered.[6] These include the frequent lack of clear, measurable program objectives. Outcome measures often do not exist and must be developed. The random assignment of patients to experimental and control or contrast groups may also present difficulties. Some of the necessary independent variables may be difficult or impossible to manipulate. Also, factors that may jeopardize the internal validity of the evaluation may be hard to control. Nevertheless, the methodological problems can often be minimized by a knowledgeable research consultant's use of research designs and processes.

Other problems encountered often fall to the manager to rectify. For example, program evaluation may be resisted by the staff. The attention evaluation research focuses on issues such as accountability, effectiveness, and efficiency can create anxiety about such matters as job security, the department's status, and one's professional reputation. If evaluation can be viewed as part of the continual treatment programming and can address questions staff want answered, it is likely to encounter little resistance. If instead, evaluation is a one-time-only effort that is forced on staff, little cooperation and use of results may follow.

SUMMARY AND CONCLUSIONS

Occupational therapists are facing escalating demands to demonstrate effectiveness and efficiency of their services. Program evaluation research is one tool that will allow occupational therapy to demonstrate its value. Additionally, therapists can receive feedback necessary to improve services. Although each evaluation must be tailored to particular needs, published reports that share measuring instruments and treatment approaches found to be effective and efficient can contribute to the knowledge building process in occupational therapy.

Program evaluation research can be an essential administrative tool that provides data for planning and policy development. When evaluation is used as a continual part of programming, it can give a systems view of a department or service. The interrelated sub-units can be viewed as to their efficiency and effectiveness.[4] The systems view is then the basis of long-range planning. Alternatives can be specified and compared as a basis for managerial decision-making. Rather than waiting and having evaluation forced on us, occupational therapy administrators should begin to develop evaluation strategies as part of treatment programming. The American Occupational Therapy Association could assist administrators by compiling a roster of qualified program evaluators. Accountability in health care is here to stay, yet a question remains about whether we have adequate data to demonstrate the worth of our services. Evaluation research can provide that data.

REFERENCES

1. Baum C: Negotiating the environment: Achieving quality care in a time of flux. *Am J Occup Ther* 36: 779-781, 1982

2. Joe B: Efficacy data project. *Am J Occup Ther* 37: 731-734, 1983

3. Green R, Attkisson C: Quality assurance and program evaluation: Similarities and differences. *Am Beh Scientist* 27:552-582, 1984

4. Biggerstaff M: The administrator and social agency evaluation. *Admin in Social Work* 1: 71-78, 1977

5. Bigman S: Evaluating the effectiveness of religious programs. *Rev of Religious Research* 2: 99, 1961

6. Grinnell R: *Social Work Research and Evaluation,* Itasca, IL: Peacock, 1985

7. Weiss C: *Evaluation Research: Methods of Assessing Program Effectiveness,* Englewood Cliffs NJ: Prentice-Hall, 1972

8. Scriven M: An introduction to meta-evaluation. *Educ Product Report* 2: 36-38, 1969

9. Suchman E: *Evaluative Research: Principles and Practice in Public Service and Action Programs,* New York: Russell Sage Foundation, 1967

10. Guttentag M, Struening E: *Handbook of Evaluation Research, Volumes I and II,* Beverly Hills: Sage, 1975

11. Tripodi T, Fellin P, Epstein I: *Differential Social Program Evaluation,* Itasca, IL: Peacock, 1978

12. Andamo E: *Guide to Program Evaluation for Physical Therapy and Occupational Therapy Services,* New York: The Haworth Press, 1984

13. Klarman H: Application of cost-benefit analysis to the health sciences. *International J of Health Services* 4: 325-352, 1974

14. Schulberg H, Baker F: Evaluating health programs: Art and/or science? In *Program Evaluation in the Health Fields,* H Schulberg, F Baker, Editors. New York: Human Sciences Press, 1979

15. Chovil A, Jacobs P: A guide to conducting an economic evaluation of an occupational health program. *Occup Health Nursing* 31: 37-40, 1983

Field Test Manual
for Prevocational Assessment

Jane T. Herrick, OTR
Helen E. Lowe, OTR

The Adult Skills Evaluation Survey for Persons with Mental Retardation (ASES) (Figure 1) is now being nationally distributed to occupational therapists and other professionals. This functional assessment identifies performance skills in adults with mild to moderate retardation. The four domains of fine motor skills, perceptual ability, academic achievement and independent living skills predict potential function in a vocationally oriented program. The manual includes the list of test materials, instructions for administration and scoring, pertinent record sheets and completed samples. The ASES is easily administered and scored.

The Adult Skills Evaluation Survey meets the need for information on performance levels of clients in a work training program. It offers significant data useful for individual program planning and effective therapy. Performance data in the manual include a graph on 84 clients tested over a four year period and a chart of performance relationships on 52 clients evaluated in 1983. The ASES was described in the journal, *Occupational Therapy in Health Care*, Volume 1, Number 2.

This article appears jointly in *Work-Related Programs in Occupational Therapy* (The Haworth Press, 1985) and *Occupational Therapy in Health Care*, Volume 2, Number 4 (Winter 1985).

113

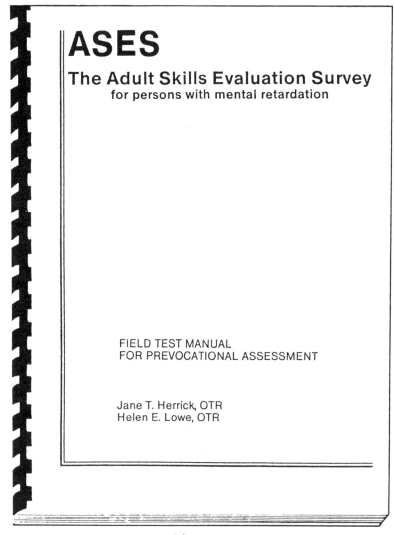

Figure 1

Testing is currently progressing to determine the reliability and validity of the instrument as a functional assessment in the work oriented environment. A critique of the field test manual is being conducted by raters on an evaluation survey which is included in the manual. Also, an evaluation sheet is disseminated to work training facilities to assess the relative importance of factors involved in successful client adaptation to the work situation.

SUMMARY

The value of functional assessments measuring dynamic characteristics of individuals within their environment is receiving increased attention in literature dealing with the adult retarded population. Occupational Therapists in this field benefit from obtaining a profile of client strengths and weaknesses related to functional abilities from which intervention can follow. It is expected that vocational readiness training will enhance the developmentally disabled individual's quality of life.

Ultimately, the availability of this instrument may improve health care delivery to persons with mental retardation through refinement of occupational therapy practice.

For further information contact Helen E. Lowe, 130 N. Fair Oaks Avenue, Pasadena, CA 91103; (818)449-0969.

BOOK REVIEWS

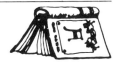

PROACTIVE VOCATIONAL HABILITATION, by Eric H. Rudrud, John P. Ziarnik, Gail S. Bernstein, Joseph M. Ferrara. *Published by Paul H. Brookes Publishing Co., P.O. Box 10624, Baltimore, MD 21204. 188pp, 1984, $15.95.*

Proactive Vocational Habilitation presents, in a well organized and easily readable form, a plan for training adults with handicapping conditions for jobs in their communities. It is based on the assumption that "competitive employment is a realistic goal for most persons currently receiving vocational habilitation and day training services," although under present systems few actually achieve such a goal. The book's intended audience consists of "persons responsible for designing and/or providing vocational habilitation services to adults with handicapping conditions." The authors' experience is predominantly with adults with mental retardation.

The contents are subdivided into four units. Each unit is comprised of chapters with objectives outlined at the beginning and with exercises and examples to illustrate the material presented.

Unit I states the philosophy of proactive habilitation, namely that it anticipates and prevents problems by training in and strengthening desired behaviors. Client goals are focused on the acquisition of adaptive skills that relate to ultimate independent functioning in "socially valid situations." In other words, the proactive approach trains people in the skills they will need to survive in work situations, preparing specifically for jobs which have been identified in their communities through "community referencing." A community referenced program establishes and maintains regular contact with employers in the community who have jobs available and are willing to employ people with disabilities. Programs in South Dakota and Colorado are cited as examples.

Unit II reviews several types of employment-directed service delivery models and how each addresses the ultimate goal of survival in a community job. Strengths and weaknesses of each type are cited. Unit III is devoted to vocational evaluations of various types and builds a rationale for a community-referenced vocational assessment program. Unit IV covers the development of a curriculum to teach work survival skills.

The philosophy of this book, in its emphasis on teaching relevant skills for daily survival, teaching them within their natural context, and teaching step by step based on careful task analysis will sound familiar to occupational therapists. While this book is specific to work situations, occupational therapists have used these same principles effectively in teaching leisure and daily living skills. With occupational therapy services likely to move increasingly into the community in the future, community referencing is a principle that could prove extremely relevant. Contacts with real situations in the real community are helpful for developmentally disabled persons served by occupational therapists, not only in vocational activities but in leisure and daily living situations as well. I would recommend this book's concrete, down-to-earth approach to colleagues who provide services for the developmentally disabled population.

Stephanie Day, MA, OTR

INTEGRATION OF DEVELOPMENTALLY DISABLED IN-DIVIDUALS INTO THE COMMUNITY. Edited by Angela R. Novak and Laird W. Heal. *Paul H. Brookes Publishers, P.O. Box 10624, Baltimore, MD 21204. 1980, 239pp, $13.95.*

This book is a significant resource in studying community placement of persons with mental retardation during the last 25 years. It includes a good history of the movement, a discussion of factors affecting positive results in integration, a perspective for future research and measures to improve the success rate of deinstitutionalization.

A number of factors pertinent to progress in community placement of persons with mental handicaps are discussed including the value of pre-release training, the importance of a comprehensive system of community services, and the need for environmental support systems. Occupational therapy is not mentioned as a habilitation factor in this book. This is unfortunate as the principles of purposeful activity, the need for assessment, the focus on activities of daily living and the concern for lessened dependency are stated as vital to successful placement. These are all central concerns for occupational therapists working with this population.

The epilogue provides a thought-provoking concept of the basic needs of deinstitutionalized persons. The authors suggest that the community must be taught to accept the handicapped person on the basis of his assets rather than deficits to allow participation as a valued member of the community.

While the many references throughout the book are valuable, their significance is diminished by the lack of current information. In a field which has shown extensive change due to legislative factors, a publication date of 1980 is a limitation. The text is useful however to document the background of the deinstitutionalization movement but it does not present a clear view of the present situation. Sylvia Bercovici, in *Barriers to Normalization, the Restrictive Management of Retarded Persons,* 1983, Baltimore: University Press, gives a more current perspective on the problems of persons with retardation in the community. Both books are helpful for a comprehensive research of the field.

Jane T. Herrick, OTR

PREVOCATIONAL AND VOCATIONAL EDUCATION FOR SPECIAL NEEDS YOUTH: A BLUEPRINT FOR THE 1980's. Edited by Kevin P. Lynch, William E. Kiernan, Jack A. Stark. *Paul H. Brookes Publishing Co., P.O. Box 10624, Baltimore, MD 21204. 305pp, 1982, $17.95.*

Occupational therapists working in the field of assessment and programming for persons who have special educational and employment needs will be pleased to discover this "blueprint" for habilitation through vocational training. The text is divided into four parts, each one presenting the contribution of several authors experienced in the implementation of services to the handicapped and the integration of special education with community programs.

An informative, historical perspective on vocational evaluation and habilitation introduces the reader to this stimulating collection of writings that address the adolescent and adult who are so often ignored in our disabled population. The 1800's saw the initial awareness of the need for vocational education for "feebleminded" children. Now in the 1980's, techniques are here for training the mentally retarded to learn skills once considered too difficult, to make changes in behavior patterns, and to prepare for positive adult work experiences. Most recently, the move to develop simulated work programs as part of secondary-level services within school systems offers new opportunities for handicapped students in their transition to the adult world of productivity and independence.

The theme throughout the book is the importance of focusing training on community-relevant vocational and social survival skills in schools and workshops. Persons with mental retardation can become vocationally competent when the training experiences are appropriate to their levels of ability. Skill acquisition and competence are critical if the handicapped are to be accepted by society. The central message is that our educational system must be integrated with the demands of the individual's environment in order to develop behaviors for success and bring about improvement in adaptation. Readers are challenged to question whether students with developmental disabilities are having the opportunity to learn the necessary skills for their future lives in community group homes and sheltered work centers.

This is a "hard-to-put-down" volume for therapists and educators who have experienced barriers to effective services for persons with learning disabilities, mental retardation, cerebral palsy and autism. It is encouraging to be challenged with current moves toward individualization in education and habilitation through effective assessment. As accentuating deficiencies stereotypes trainees as non-useful, with little chance for advancement, so building on acquired abilities is the promising area of growth in prevocational settings. All the sections of the book direct attention to the appropriate evaluating of individual skills, teaching how to apply those skills and concepts, and then generalizing them to the workshop environment. The writers applaud progress in secondary-level services, research in biomedical techniques and improved sociological attitudes.

Unfortunately, although there is a chapter on cerebral palsy written by an occupational therapist, there is no recognition in the book of the role occupational therapy should play in the continuum of vocational preparation in the school to the treatment oriented program in the community based setting. However, the many in our profession who are dealing with the underevaluation of our role in vocational readiness for persons with developmental incapacity can value this text as a stimulus to designing and implementing models of service delivery that are in keeping with our identity and basic interest in the holistic, comprehensive improvement of task performance.

Helen E. Lowe, OTR

FUNCTIONAL ASSESSMENT IN REHABILITATION. Edited by Andrew S. Halpern and Marcus J. Fuhrer. *Paul H. Brookes Publishing Company, P.O. Box 10624, Baltimore, MD 21204. 1984, 272pp, $23.95.*

This text is a comprehensive and scholarly review and documentation of the current status of 'functional assessment' in rehabilitation. It traces the politics, describes the many differences and changes that have occurred in rehabilitation philosophies, explains the complexities and problems involved in rehabilitation assessments and suggests resolutions to problems. The fifteen chapters in the book represent the research and work of professionals from many disciplines, including occupational therapy, and from institutions located in 13 of the United States. The contributors initially develop new insights for defining 'functional assessment'. They further describe procedures required to administer 'functional assessments' correctly, give descriptions of some exemplary instruments as well as suggestions for different uses of the information gleaned from assessment. Each author presents a thesis for applying functional assessment to: identifying patient needs, choosing appropriate service interventions, monitoring responses to treatment and evaluating service outcomes in order to document program accountability. 'Functional assessment' was applied to the different needs for assessment found in various fields of rehabilitation, including physical and psychiatric restoration, mental retardation and communication disorders.

Importantly, the book offers the reader many diverse options to use in gathering assessment information. Interviews, question-naires, self-reports, rating scales, tests, direct observations, simulations (role play), technical devices and examination of historical documents are all available alternatives to traditional standardized test procedures.

The key theme of the book is to define and compare 'functional assessment' to 'traditional rehabilitation assessment'. The early concept of rehabilitation as reflected in *traditional assessment procedures* was based on a pathology-oriented view of the individual and a reductionist concern for the bits and pieces of effects from an impairment or disorder. Medical rehabilitation, then is seen as generally a long term effort to alleviate impairments, maintain health status and preserve or restore behavioral functioning. Current views of rehabilitation as embodied in 'functional assessment' approaches, on the other hand, presumably address problems of environmental interactions, focus on the individual's adaptive processes and are concerned with the person's ability to resume roles, rights and responsibilities for a satisfying daily life and community involvement.

Therefore, *functional assessment* is described as a behavioral approach based upon a psychosocial model which measures the individual's responses to particular life situations and his or her interactions with the surrounding environment. This 'newer' viewpoint is compatible with the bio-psycho-social frame of reference inherent in current occupational therapy practice.

Finally, the text is of value to vocational rehabilitation and health care professionals concerned with assisting disabled individuals to achieve the fullest physical, mental, social, vocational and economic usefulness for which they are capable. The authors have integrated their knowledge into a comprehensive perspective of rehabilitation and have conveyed new ways of thinking about assessment which reflect the current state of the art within their field. Thereby the book is not only a valuable reference to those working directly with patients and clients but a useful tool for those involved with future developments in rehabilitation research.

Janith McCready Hurff, MA, OTR

OCCUPATIONAL THERAPY: WORK-RELATED PROGRAMS AND ASSESSMENTS. Karen Jacobs. *Little, Brown and Company, Boston, Massachusetts, 02106. 1985, 286pp.*

This work is a welcome addition to the limited current information for occupational therapists in the area of work-related programming. The focus of this book is to provide the reader with information helpful in designing and implementing work-related programs and assessments. It should be noted that the author selected the term work-related as opposed to the terms prevocational or vocational because she felt these terms were derived from other professions and that the term work-related is occupational therapy terminology.

The book contains six chapters, beginning with the history of work-related programs in occupational therapy and ending with future considerations. Chapter 1 provides light and useful information on the history of occupational therapy's involvement in prevocational and vocational activities. The second chapter deals with establishing a conceptual framework. The author feels that work-related programming is a holistic and life span process. She indicates that work-related activities should not be initiated during adolescence or adulthood but should be occurring throughout the life span. This chapter briefly discusses traditional standardized and nonstandardized evaluations and provides a basis for the development of the author's own evaluation instrument. The author provides a detailed description of the Jacobs Prevocational Skills Assessment in the following chapter. This assessment was developed for a learning-disabled adolescent population. Included are task descriptions, forms, and other graphics that may be reproduced by readers for their own clinical use.

Jacobs also includes chapters describing various work-related programs for children and adults in this country, Canada, and Australia. Although the material is not as extensive as the material on the author's own programs it provides helpful descriptions dealing with programs for persons in a variety of diagnostic groups in assorted settings. The author offers descriptions of work-related programs for individuals with psychosocial problems, neurophysiologic problems, the developmentally disabled, and the traumatically injured. She concludes by offering material on future considerations such as the use of computers in work-related programming.

Occupational Therapy: Work-Related Programs and Assessments is a welcome addition to the profession's current body of knowledge. The style of this work fosters easy and understandable reading. The task descriptions, forms, and graphics included for the Jacobs Prevocational Skills Assessment provide the reader with clear guidelines for administering that assessment. This book would be a helpful resource for students and practicing occupational therapists interested in obtaining information on work-related programming.

Kathy Reynolds-Lynch, OTR

MANAGEMENT AND PRINCIPLES FOR HEALTH PROFESSIONS. Joan G. Liebler, Ruth E. Levine, and Hyman L. Dervitz. *Aspen Publications, Aspen Systems Corp., 1600 Research Blvd., Rockville, MD 20850. 1984, 339pp, $33.00.*

''The work of health care . . . demands much from the health care practitioner, who must balance the science of management with the art of human relations.'' This thesis forms the focus in this text for this trio of authors from differing health professions. The work summarizes in a clear, logical manner the scholarly substance of several basic M.B.A. management courses.

Though the theory and application of management theme is common to countless books, the authors primarily tailor their extensive coverage of the development of management theory to the manner in which it applies to practical situations for professionals such as occupational therapists, physical therapists and medical records administrators. The case studies and the examples are found sprinkled throughout each chapter, although only the chapter on MBO (Management by Objectives) has considerable depth and detail to assure the understanding by the would-be-manager.

Management and Principles for Health Professions clearly summarizes with well-documented, classic, management references the many theories and applications of its topic. Its chapters are well organized and written with a consistent style, though the book's character is dry and technical to read. The information presented is of great value to new health managers as a departmental and personal resource, but the book's tepid tone requires a certain amount of discipline on the part of the reader to continue. Further, it falls short of fully modeling the importance of a leadership personality for the aspiring manager though it does arm one with complete management information.

Mary M. Evert, MBA, OTR, FAOTA